Welcome to New Orleans....
How many shots did you HEAR?

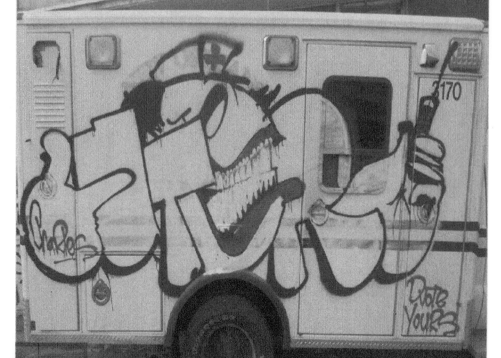

True stories working as a medic and a cop in and around the Big Easy

B.J. Schneider NRP COSM

Other Books by B.J. Schneider:

Fiction

A Salty Life & A Traitor's Death (A Hannibal Greco Novel)

Non-Fiction

Welcome to New Orleans Volume 2… The Life you saved may take your own.

A Taste of The Big Easy — [signature]

WELCOME TO NEW ORLEANS... HOW MANY SHOTS DID YOU HEAR?

By: B.J. Schneider NRP COSM

Copyright 2015 XIPHOS BOOKS

Copyright© 2015 by XIPHOS BOOKS

Second edition 2016 XIPHOS BOOOKS

All rights reserved.

No part of this book may be reproduced or retransmitted in any form or by any means without the written permission of the publisher.

Published by Xiphos Books

This is a work of the author's memory and impressions. Names, characters, places, and incidents are the product of the author's feeble mind. Any resemblance to actual persons, living or dead, events, or locales are entirely coincidental.

For more information, visit
www.xiphosbooks.net

Dedication

I wish to dedicate this book to my wife Rose and my kids Brittanie and Blade. They are the reasons my sanity survived all these years.

I would also like to dedicate this book to all the men and women of EMS that are out there every day dedicating their lives to saving others.

PREFACE

Welcome to New Orleans. We'll try and keep the gunfire to a minimum. This collection of short stories is a mix of some of the more interesting moments of my years working the streets as both a Paramedic and on occasion a cop.

If I have done my job, these peeks into my world will take you on a ride of emotions. I want you to laugh out loud, and yes, if I can make you sniffle and choke up a bit, I would be ecstatic.

This book has no chapters, this is odd but I swear I have a reason, and I hope you agree. In EMS you have no idea what the next call will be. Is it a silly drunk or the end results of a gunfight? All are possible, but you'll have to turn on the lights and sirens and get moving to see what's around the next corner. To let you travel with us the stories are laid out in no particular order with no chapters so each story, each call, is a surprise in your journey.

The title of this book comes from a time in the city when murders were at a record high and the number of ambulances working the streets were at an all-time low. The city of New Orleans Health Department had six fulltime trucks around the clock and two additional units for high volume hours. This was in a city of 750,000 residences plus the hundreds of thousands that came to work and play from outside the city limits.

It was not unusual for a unit to respond to 20 calls in a 12-hour shift and to have several of those be gun or knife related. Tourism of course suffered and so did the tourists. So the running gag was "Welcome to New Orleans. How many shots did you hear?" Which was the line asked of all your shooting victims to gauge how many holes they might have in them. It is only funny in the sense that the volume of violence we were dealing with caused our humor to be dark just to cope.

Some of the stories that follow are funny yes, but you may find yourself laughing and thinking why am I laughing at this? It's like staring at a car accident. You don't want to stare but you can't tear your eyes away. Its okay it's only natural, trust me I'm a professional.

I must take a moment to tell you that these are my stories, written from my memories for whatever that's worth. They are true to the best of my knowledge but to quote a friend of mind I'm not going to let the truth get in the way of a good story.

So, sit back, get your latex gloves on, and prepare to get a little messy. It's Saturday night in New Orleans and the full moon is up. It's gonna be a crazy one!

TO PEE OR NOT TO PEE

Some days, life as a paramedic in a big city, can be busy. I mean REALLY busy. This, in and of itself, isn't a problem. You learn to roll with the punches. Missed meals, or meals on the move, no breaks, or time to relax. You just run from call to call to call. The dispatchers are begging and pleading with you to leave wherever you are to go to somewhere else. None of this is truly a new problem but, as the old saying goes, when you have to go you have to go! This can be a problem compounded by having a partner that has a highly refined sense of bathroom humor.

We had a cardiac arrest call. Extremely taxing on both mind and body but on this Saturday there was no rest for the wicked. We hadn't even changed the sheets on the gurney when dispatch was calling us reporting a 34S. That, to the uninitiated is Louisiana state code slang. 34 for Aggravated Assault, S for shooting. This is the drug of the 911 medic. A call for a shooting is the adrenalin pumper we live for.

As you can imagine, we said sure, we got it. We crammed the stretcher back in the unit and poured on gasoline and sirens heading for the call.

The one thing I had forgotten in the rush for my trauma call fix was that I had to piss. I mean bad. There was no way in hell I was going to be able to do all the acrobatic lifting, strapping, bandaging and IV work without peeing down my leg. Thankfully we were slobs and had left over sports drink bottles and junk in the front of the truck cab.

I slid forward on the seat to kneel in the front well of the truck figuring this would give me the best degree of control and privacy. This plan was sound except for one small flaw. The maniacal guy driving the unit.

Raymond "Mad Dog" Mandola was an excellent paramedic, a good partner and an evil no good fucker. If he thought there was a joke to be had with any degree of malice. As long as it was aimed at you he had no problem taking the jab. He saw that I was kneeling in the front well, hands down low holding the bottle and aiming.

This presented a unique opportunity to abuse me. We were traveling down Interstate 10 at 70 plus MPH. He waited until he made eye contact with me then grinned this grin that would have disturbed the Cheshire cat..........

Brake!!

Accelerate!!

Brake!!!

Accelerate!!!

This was his plot. As he tapped the brake my head was thrown forward. I had a split second choice, which really is no choice at all. Do I let go of the bottle and piss down my leg, so that I could reach up and protect myself......or.......lower my head and take the face to the windshield?

I opted (reluctantly) for door number 2.

WHACK! My face slammed into the glass for a split second then he hits the gas again throwing me back. Before I could find balance, brake! Face to glass again.

This went on for several miles of interstate while he cackled in gales of laughter and I cursed and sputtered and tried not to pee on myself.

This is a warning tale of evil friends and poor timing. Remember that your friends are just moments from doing you harm as long as they feel it's funny.

~~EGGPLANT LADY~~ 〜〜〜〜〜〜〜〜〜〜〜〜〜〜〜〜〜〜〜〜〜〜〜〜〜

Some calls let you know really early that they are going to be bad. So you need to look, listen (and smell) the warning signs.

It's July in the Big Easy. That's bad for a few reasons. The first is obvious…..it's hot….Africa hot….crotch hot. It's a level of hot that changes people's mental faculties.

Dispatch called our unit with a possible 29S. That's Louisiana radio code for a possible suicide. The address given was a third floor apartment (of course) in the French Quarter. This was starting out poorly.

We pull up in front of the address and see that both NOPD (2 cars) and our own supervisor are already on the scene.

The supervisor on the scene is C.J., an old salt with a wicked sense of gallows humor. I called him on the radio as we got out asking what equipment we needed. His response was a chuckle followed by, clipboard only. With that bit of information we started up the old stair case. We met C.J. on the second floor landing. He was heading down as we were heading up. He was laughing and shaking his head. His only comment as he passed us was "Smell you later." This should have been clue #1.

Clue #2 came as soon as we made the third floor landing. There was a window on the landing that overlooked a court yard. The window was open and an NOPD officer was leaning out of it vomiting his guts into the court yard below. Oh shit this was going to be bad……

The building obviously did not have air conditioning. The smell was wafting from the open apartment door on to the third floor landing. It was a smell that all cops and medics eventually know, never forget, and loath to the core of their souls. Death. Rot. It is hard to describe. Its meat gone bad, times one hundred, but it's mixed with something no other animal possesses. It's a smell unique to the death of humans alone.

I took as deep a breath as I could and entered. There was a French Settee, kind of like a love seat, in the middle of the single room apartment. On the sofa was what remained of a very heavy set woman who in life had long bleach blonde hair.

She had been dead for three days. I can say this with certainty because she had left one of the most detailed suicide notes I had ever read. She had laid out the letter on a stool next to her body and included her driver's license for identification. The letter stated that she had been depressed and tired of living. It explained in a very dispassionate way that she had bought a large amount of heroin and was going to inject it in herself. It was all very clinical.

The problem which she could never have imagined is that her lack of close friendships and relations had not only assisted in her depression but complicated her demise. She had laid in this room with no ventilation in the middle of July. The gases in her body had caused her to bloat. The heat and rot had blackened her skin until it had a purple sheen. Her bleached hair protruded from her swollen body like the dried stem of a giant eggplant. It was bizarre and horrific all at the same time.

The second problem with July is that last year's medical students graduated at the end of May and they are now Doctors. These brand new doctors are now Interns and begin their first rotations in the Emergency Room.

As with all deaths in New Orleans they aren't dead until a doctor has officially declared them dead. All medics understand that this is a formality. We are there with our eyes and other senses on the person. The doctors via phone or radio must have trust in the medics at the other end of the line and the medics must be clear and concise in the telling of the information. July creates a problem because the doctors are brand new and shiny. Still wet behind the ears and not knowing the medics. They barely know the "by the book" aspect of their job. This causes some communication issues.

I called Charity Hospital on the radio and got a baby doc that I had to tell to push the button to talk and release to listen....sigh....this was going to be difficult. "Doc I have a 27 year old white female. She is pulseless and apneic. She has been deceased three days and is extremely bloated, discolored and disfigured. I am requesting a DNR (Do not Resuscitate) and a time of death." Doc's response is a little disconcerting. "Did you run an EKG?"

Now you must understand that this whole conversation is going on from the landing as far away from the body as I can get without fleeing the building. In an effort to keep from being an outright liar I pretend I didn't hear his question and simply repeat my entire report. He asks the question again......... A lot of thoughts go through my mind at that moment. Is he serious? If I lie I could get in trouble. If I tell the truth I'll have to go place EKG leads on her bloated oozing......that does it!..."Doc EKG shows asystole in all three leads.....did I mention she is bloated and oozing like over ripe fruit?"......."DNR granted"

With that bit of business out of the way I was working on the report. While I finished up the Coroner's Office arrived. This consisted of one overworked civil servant and two prisoners on work release. This must have been the time of year for new prisoners too because these two guys looked clueless.

The Coroner's guy came over to shoot the shit with me and sent his workers to bag up the body. As I was writing the report and talking I was watching over his shoulder at the guys trying to load the body into the body bag. The way to do this would be to wrap the body in the bag and close it up. This was not what they were doing.

These guys had placed the bag on the floor in front of the Settee and as if in slow motion I realized what they were going to do and couldn't stop them. They both reached out and grabbed this unfortunate women's body and tried to roll it off the love seat to the bag on the floor. I yelled to stop but it was too late. The body struck the hard wood floor and after days of putrefaction it was mostly liquefied inside the soft skin. When it struck it was like the largest, grossest water balloon in the world had exploded. The body ruptured and sprayed both of the prisoners in a layer of black bodily fluids that made everyone around gag.

I grabbed my clip board and started to flee down the stairs. The last thing I saw and heard was one of the prisoners standing rigid with his hands out in front of his face. The only thing I could hear was him repeating NO. NO, NO, NO, NO NO.............

I hope he got credit for time served.

GINGER'S FIRST DAY

I've always considered myself prompt. The Army drilled into me that if I wasn't early, I was late. So, arriving for my night shift late was frustrating and embarrassing. To make matters worse my supervisor, E.J., was standing at the bay doors of the station grinning at me as I walked up.

As I approached he said it looked like I was having a little trouble. I told him I was, and apologized for being tardy. He blew it off and told me that my regular partner was sent out on a call, so he was putting me with someone else.

"Who?"

His grin turned into a large smile.

"Fred."

"NO!"

"Oh yea."

Fred was a paramedic that had joined our ranks just weeks earlier from somewhere out west. He was already making a name for himself as a bumbling idiot. Him as my partner was my punishment for being late.

"I'll try and soften the blow. I have a third rider, a new volunteer, I'll put with you to help out." E.J. dead panned.

I didn't trust E.J. he was having too much fun. "What's the catch?"

"Tonight is her first shift with us."

Now having a third rider can be helpful, because it's an extra set of hands and can make for an easier shift. Even someone that had never worked with us could be useful although they wouldn't know our way of doing things.

"OK, where is he at?"

"She."

"She?"

E.J. pointed into the bay toward where I saw Fred milling about. Ginger was a very cute girl that couldn't be 95 pounds if I hosed her down and put rocks in her pockets. Maybe 5 foot tall at a stretch.

I walked up, told Fred to load the truck, and introduced myself to Ginger. We grabbed the rest of the gear and headed to the truck.

Me: "So, E.J. tells me this is your first shift working with us correct?"

Ginger: "Yes, this is my first time. I just got my EMT-Basic."

Me: "So how much experience have you had?"

Ginger: "This is my first time."

Me: "With us. Right?"

Ginger: "First time on an ambulance'"

Oh mother of all that is holy!!

Me: "Hmmm...OK, well keep your eyes open, listen to what's going on and don't hesitate to ask me questions. If I don't answer it immediately it's probably because I'm busy. We will get to it as soon as I can. Oh, and one last thing, don't listen to anything Fred says................"

No sooner were we loaded in the truck dispatch assigns us to a cardiac arrest in a nearby Italian restaurant......crap

I drive. Fred drums the dashboard like he's auditioning for Motley Crue. Ginger peers forward from the back of the truck with a deer in the headlights look.

We pull up and headed inside, it is definitely a cardiac arrest and CPR is being performed. We have a good news/ bad news situation.

The good news is there are several doctors in the restaurant and they have started CPR.

The bad news is there are several doctors in the restaurant and they are arguing over proper care of the recent recipient of the Osso Bucco.

OK, I am the senior medic on the truck so it's my job to run this goat rodeo.

"You doctor spaghetti on your shirt, yes you, keep doing CPR."

"Fred, get him on the monitor see what we have to work with."

"I'll start airway. Ginger, go to the truck and get a spine board."

Ginger takes two steps and stops. I knew at that very moment that she would make an excellent medic. She only took two steps. Then she turned and asked "Where in the truck?"

"Side cabinet looks like an outhouse door. Go, go, go!"

I've gotten him intubated at this point. Fred has him on the monitor and it's V-Fib, ventricular fibrillation. This is a rhythm that needs shocking.

Fred charges the paddles and calls clear, then he does the most bizarre thing I think I've ever seen. He yells "BAM!" as he discharges the shock into the patient. Still V-fib, charge for another shock. He yells "RIDE THE LIGHTING!"

One of the doctors makes eye contact with me and I make a face that says "I have no idea what he is doing."

I've gotten an IV started, got the first round of drugs on board as Ginger makes it back with a spine board, just a spine board, no straps, no tape, but a very nice spine board. I was just about to explode at her when I realized that A) It was her first day on a truck, and B) She brought me exactly what I asked for....I guess I should have been clearer.

We get him on the spine board Fred makes one more inappropriate utterance to the crowd and shocks the patient again and we are off to the truck. The Patient is sliding off the spine board and trying to fall off the stretcher, since we had nothing to secure him with.

We get him in the truck and miracle of miracles we have gotten a heart beat back on our patient! I have Fred and Ginger (yea I know I didn't think about the names until years later) secure him to the board and continue to ventilate him as I set up maintenance drip of medication.

I have come to a very difficult point in this call. Fred is new to New Orleans, and nuttier than a Christmas fruit cake. Can I trust him to find the hospital if I let him drive? The other choice is I put poor ginger in the back with him and drive as fast as humanly possible hoping that he doesn't kill the patient as I make my way to the E.R.

"Fred?" "Yea?"

"Do you know how to get to Mercy Hospital from here?"

He actually pauses and looks out the window. "Sort of?" "Well I know its back in the direction we came from."

Although technically correct his answer did not build confidence in his navigating abilities. "I'll drive Fred. You just monitor his vitals."

"Ginger, just keep ventilating him you're doing good."

I scamper to the front of the truck and head with reckless abandon toward the hospital figuring the longer Fred is back there the less chance the patient has and the greater chance that Ginger will be scarred for life.

We make it to the E.R. and pass our patient off for care. Afterward, we are outside putting the truck back together and showing Ginger that spine boards actual come with straps. She stops me and asks "Is it always like this?"

I sigh and look at her. "Only when I'm late for work."

NOTIFICATION

Its Thanksgiving week. There was an accident. A head on collision, on a two lane highway. A man decided to commit suicide by crossing the center line. He went head on with a minivan and killed a Vietnamese couple in the van as well as himself. We are on the scene with a State Trooper and have had to call our medical control and pronounce all three people deceased.

The Trooper looks pissed. I walk over to give him some information and see what's bothering him. As we talk he tells me that as he has gotten more information on all our victims, he has found that our solo driver that crossed the center line had a note in his pocket. He had been recently arrested and was out on bail and knew he was going to prison so he took his life. The Trooper nearly spits these words as he says them. "Fucker didn't seem to care about the people he rammed into."

Timing being what it is the family of the couple that was killed took this moment to show up on scene. It was as horrible and disturbing as you can imagine. We had to physically carry them away from the vehicles seeing up close the pain and misery they were experiencing.

By the time we had removed the bodies and the trooper had finished his investigation several hours had passed and to say that the Trooper was fuming would be an understatement. He was seething as he walked around and kept mumbling under his breath. I wouldn't want to be the one that would incur his wrath.

As we were preparing to leave the Trooper came to ask me a favor. He said he was going to make notification, meaning he was going to the residence of our suicide guy and tell his family that he was dead. I told him we would head out with him just in case we were needed. To myself I thought "Well this should be interesting!"

We follow the Trooper to the home address of our dead suicide king and let the Trooper take the lead at the door. He straightens his hat and knocks on the door.

A women in her fifties answers the door she has a cigarette burning in one hand and a tall boy beer in the other. She looks right up at the Trooper and says "What in hell does the Poe-lease want at my house?" The Troopers back visibly stiffens at this. He looks down his nose at her and asks in his deep commanding voice.

"Do you have a son that drives a 78 Chevy Nova?"

"Yea that's my boy. What of it?" she says.

"Did he leave here earlier wearing jeans and a plaid shirt?"

"That's how he was dressed. What kinda thing ya'll tryin to pin on'um now?" she harshly responds.

The Trooper pauses for a long moment to control the anger you can see boiling just under the surface.

His next question seems somewhat off topic.

"How many people will you be at your table for Thanksgiving?"

The women looks at him equally as confused as we are. She finally says seven people will be at Thanksgiving dinner.

In a dead pan voice, the Trooper looks right at her and says "You can pick one of those place setting up. Juniors dead."

My jaw falls open. My partners jaw falls open. The women faints and falls back onto the floor.

The Trooper does and about face and heads to his car. He finally looks at me and asks "You got this?" I can do nothing but stare since I cannot find the words.

FIRST NIGHT

I considered myself a fairly experienced medic. I had been in the army, worked as a cop and had been a medic for a 9-1-1 service in the suburbs for years. Despite this experience, I'm not sure if it prepared me for my first night at in the city of New Orleans.

I was working the 7pm to 7am shift and was assigned my partner Bill. Bill defined the term larger than life, He was 6 foot 5 at least and had to top the scales at 400 pounds. These things alone were not the only things that made him stand out. Bill had a lazy eye and loved strippers. An interesting combination I know. It made him a very interesting first partner.

It was a Monday night and after midnight things had finally slowed down. I was in Paramedic school during the day and asked Bill if I could lay in the back of the unit and study (read this as sleep). He was cool about it and said sure he was just going to run the figure eight.

Now the figure eight was a route the medics would take through the French Quarter. It optimized your view of clubs, bars and especially strip joints and that was right up Bill's alley. So off to study land I went.

I woke up in the back and something seemed wrong. It took me a minute to figure it out. First, it was hot and stuffy. The engine was off. That played right into number two. It was quiet, too quiet as a dime store drama novel would say.

I eased to the back doors and stepped out. My watch said it was 4am. I looked up at the street sign and we were parked at the bottom of the figure eight on the corner of Iberville and Charters. The truck was empty.... Where the hell was Bill???

The business in front of the truck was a strip club (shocking!!!) it was an old school New Orleans building with both walls made up of numerous French doors. Being the wee hours of the morning all the doors were open and you could look straight into the club. Oh crap.....I found my partner.

Inside the club was a pool table. The lazy eyed giant of a partner was playing pool..........with a naked women......in uniform....exposed to the world. I am so fired, and on my first day!!

I walked over to the doors closest to him and made a point not to enter. Bill looked up and smiled a shit eating grin. Looking at me and the girl...... at the same time.

He said "You wanna play with the winner?"

~~YOU ARE MY SUNSHINE~~

In the early 90s the city of New Orleans got a brand new radio system. It had lots of bells and whistles including one the medics came to enjoy called I-call. I-call was a way to dial the number of someone else's radio so you could talk one on one. A great function for passing on information but even better for causing mischief.

Darren had the evil habit of I-calling his friends and singing to them to drive them crazy. It was always very funny in private. Today it was hilariously funny for the world.

Through some unknown technical difficulty, as Darren attempted to key in his target for amusement, he keyed into the main channel where all the units were. He then began to sing.

"You are my sunshine, my only sunshine, you make me happy, when skies are gray. You'll never know dear, how much I love you............"

He serenaded the whole city of New Orleans and had no idea he was doing it. The minute he finished the cheers and cat calls over the radio were riotous. He had to be stunned. The problem was that one of his listeners was not as wowed by his musical abilities as the rest.

The Head of EMS operations got on the Radio. "Mr. (Full name hidden to protect the guilty) you and your orchestra, my office, now!!!!

~~ENCYCLOPEDIA SALESMAN OR LANGUAGE BY COMMITTEE~~

The hotels in New Orleans are a regular stop for crews. Being such a big tourist and convention city, full of people doing things they might not do back in Middle America, it was not un-common to be called to them.

My partner for this night was a good friend, Cesar. We always had fun working together because we had a high regard for the technical side of our medical work but also enjoyed goofing off during our down time. Cesar is Latino. His family is from Honduras and he is fluent in Spanish.

His ability to speak Spanish was important today because dispatch called us in need of his language skills.

Dispatch calls and says we have a guy in the security office at the Marriott that they say, appears injured but they can't understand him.

We get to the hotel and meet up with Security and our patient. Cesar spoke to him in Spanish asking him what had happened.

He starts rattling away high speed and an odd thing happened. I realize I understand some of what he was saying and I didn't speak Spanish. At the same time Cesar looks over at me with a smirk on his face. "Um….that's not Spanish. At least most of it isn't."

Well with a force of will we were able to determine that our patient was from Brazil. He spoke Portuguese. Some of the words were Spanish or close enough for Cesar to translate and being he and I were both good Catholic school boys we could work out some of the Latin based words that are a large portion of Portuguese.

The punch line of this story is what we were able to figure out happened.

Our patient was beat up while walking back to his hotel from his convention and his samples were taken from him..........His encyclopedia samples.

He was a giant cliché. A beat up encyclopedia salesman.

~~DO YOU MISS IT~~

As I talk to people about my career in EMS and then about my time away from the hustle and bustle, I am always asked the same question. Do you miss it?

I wish that was a question that was black and white, instead it needs much deeper explaining.

In my opinion 9-1-1 work, especially in New Orleans, is just like a drug addiction. The feelings you get when you're doing it is a high like no other. You're on top of the world. You feel like what you can only guess a god feels like. You chase that feeling your whole career, but for some, you finally realize that the thing you love so much is actually stealing your life away from you. It's destroying your relationships, swallowing your youth and breeding a degree of cynicism in you that can taint your life.

So you break the chain of addiction and escape. You're happier, healthier, a better partner and parent, but when the lights are out and you hear a siren off in the distance you feel a little twitch in your muscles. The siren sound is much like the mythical Siren's song drawing you toward the rocky shoals once again............... It never leaves you.

THE STREETS OF SAN FRANCISCO

I love to travel. I especially love to travel on someone else's dime. I had the great fortune to be in San Francisco to help teach a class. I also got to visit with one of my best friends, a Captain with the San Francisco EMS Department. He was kind enough to get me a day shift ride along with one of the crews working downtown S.F. I thought it would be fun, as well as a good insight to the people I'd be teaching the next days.

We had been running calls for about 4 or 5 hours and were getting lunch in the Mission District up on the hill when we got a call down in the Embarcadero at the waterfront.

Now, I'm sitting in the back of the truck in the jump seat with my hosts in the front seats. We are looking down a street that leads all the way down to the bay. It is all downhill, leveling out at each cross street.

The lead paramedic reaches up and flips all the emergency beacons on and looks back at me with an evil grin............He asks an odd and foreboding question. "Did you ever watch the TV show 'The Streets of San Francisco'?"

Before I could udder a word, the other partner turns on the siren and nails the throttle. We are heading down hill in a 7 ton brick filled with sharp objects. We hit the cross street and I can feel us compress on the shocks and then as we hit the next downhill section......WE GO AIRBORNE.......The supplies in the cabinets are not secured down; have I mentioned that?

Every time we take air, medical supplies come flying out of the cabinets, I go flying through the air, then BAM!! Everything, including me come crashing down

....over and over and over and over again. I'm having visions of Karl Malden and Michael Douglas.

We finally get to our call. The medics meet me at the back doors of the truck. I am ragged, the trucks a mess and all they say to me is "Your initiation is complete. Welcome to San Francisco EMS."

MAKE YOUR SKIN CRAWL

It goes without saying that when working as a 911 medic, you see people at their worst. What most people don't think of is that we see peoples' houses at their very worst also. Dirty, funky, and sometimes just gross, but this one takes the prize.

Its 4am. My partner and I are in the St. Thomas housing project at a call for something that has long ago faded from my memory. We walk into the back door of the apartment that enters the kitchen. It's illuminated by a black drop light. The light bulb section is hooked to the ceiling by a nail. The extension cord drapes over the stove area and hangs down to a plug on the counter.

As we move through the room, I brush the hanging black extension cord. It moved.

NO....I mean it undulated, wriggled, rippled, wobbled......holy St. Francis!!!

It's not a black extension cord! It's an orange extension cord covered in LIVE roaches. The grease from years of frying food on the stove had coated the cord and become a home for the roaches.

If you're reading this and don't have the itchy creepy crawlies, you're not human.......

~~MAKING~~ ~~FRIENDS~~ ~~AND~~ ~~BOOBY~~ ~~TRAPPING~~ ~~PEOPLE~~~~~~

As a young pup in EMS, I was able to get assigned to the Sheriff's Offices EMS/ Rescue squad. My new Lieutenant was also going to be my partner.... oh joy.

Like any new guy, I wanted to make a good impression with my new boss so I elicited aid and advice from the Sergeant, Ralph. Ralph was a crusty old bastard. The one picture that always comes to mind that describes him is seeing him hunched over in a cloud of Lucky Strike smoke half way through a solitaire game with old worn cards.

That description should give you an idea of the type of advice I got from Sarge.......

He tells me. Well Mike, the Lt., is a tough guy. He would really appreciate someone that got the best of him with a prank.

I bite. Hook, line and sinker......sigh (God, I was dumb at that age.)

Mike was big into military history, strategies and tactics, and since I had not been out of the Army for long, I'd go with a military style prank.

I massaged the lock on his office (That's a euphemism for broke in.) and once in, I did a classic booby trap. I taped a glass jar to the floor on the door knob side, loaded it with a hand grenade.

Hang on a minute....don't freak just take a deep breath. It was a training grenade. Just a dud.

I pulled the pin and slide it into the jar, tied fishing line around the neck of the grenade and secured it to the hinge of the door and sealed the office back up.

The medic's room was next to Mike's office, so I was huddled by the door listing for his arrival, listening like a parent waiting for their teenager to come home from a date.

First clue was the jingle of his keys, then the key in the lock. Oh the anticipation was killing me!!! As I hear the squeak of the door swinging open, I know its time. The sounds that follow made me think the grenade was real......

A gigantic boom (Mike's bag of books slamming into the floor), a scuttle and a crash (Mike's body flying back out the office door, then slamming into the floor), a fluttering sound (Mike's stack of papers he was carrying flying through the air).

I consider Mike one of my best friends to this day. That bonding prank was not the high point of that friendship.

PAID IN CASH

It's not uncommon when working in downtown New Orleans to be just minutes away from the Emergency Room. So the care you give and the things that happen take place in a high speed condensed window of time.

It was winter in New Orleans, all three days of it, and John and I had just gotten a call in the Lafitte Housing Project of a shooting (34S). When we arrive we find a young (20s) male laying on his back on the ground of the court yard. The rapid assessment shows 2 gunshot wounds to the chest. Being less than 2 minutes from the hospital meant that our care would be battlefield fast and only the most life threating things would be handled.

We exposed his chest, dressed the wounds, and got him on a spine board and immediately into the truck. In any school as a field medic, you are taught that a trauma patient should be a naked patient, but we knew his best chance was in the operating room, not hanging around with us in the courtyard. Time was not his friend and there was no time. We simply opened his jacket and ripped his shirt open, nothing more.

We ran the 90 second transport and got our patient to Charity hospital's trauma room (room 4). We passed our patient over to the staff and backed up to do our post call clean up and information collection. The Trauma team went about their routine which started with cutting all the patients clothes off.

A couple of nurses started at both his feet, put the scissors to the seams of his jeans and ran up to the waist. As they went through both his pockets it suddenly began raining twenty dollar bills. The stretcher, the floor, everything had cash sliding over it. My partner John and I just looked at each other for a minute and he said in a dead pan voice. "Finally one that could have paid in cash."

AMBULANCE SURFING

Medics are amazing in their heroism, their ability to work under pressure in a hostile environment, but when you live so close to the edge of the envelope you tend to make poor decisions when seeking additional thrills. This leads to a pastime of some of the more mentally feeble of us known as ambulance surfing.

It was my very last day as a Paramedic at the city of New Orleans. I was moving to a more stable, steady job.........Parole agent.....yea, I know, I was still chasing the dragon, but that's another story.

My partner for the night was Cesar, a stellar medic and a good friend. We planned on making the most out of my last night.

We started around midnight with ambulance bowling. What you say? You've never heard of this? Let me explain.

You find a closed supermarket parking lot. You round up enough shopping baskets to make a pin set up (standing them on their ends of course) with one extra. You strategically place the extra in the front of your ambulance. You then push your basket and steer your truck to knock down the others....Simple. We started getting board since we could seem to make a strike and wanton destruction of private property had gotten old fairly quickly. Time for something else......Next.

Cesar: "So what do you wanna do?"

Me: "Something that will get me fired?"

Cesar: "That's pretty much anything you do most shifts."

ME: "Fuck off"

Cesar: "How about one more surf?"

Me: "Outstanding idea"

Cesar: "Out-FREAKING-standing!"

So how this works is your partner picks a road, preferably a long straight road, and gets up to a nice cruising speed. You, in this case me, climbs out of the passenger window and maneuvers up on to the roof. You get up to your feet in a classic Laird Hamilton pose and holler to your partner to hit it.

This would be the point when they turn on all the lights and sirens and pick up speed racing down the road. This tends to draw stares from pedestrians and wide eyed panicked looks from other motorists.

Is this dangerous?......................YES

Is this kind of juvenile?..............Yep

Is it a rush that an adrenal junkie like me couldn't help but partake in?

Damn Skippy!!

MARDI GRAS GONE BAD

Mardi Gras, an amazing time for locals and visitors alike, but some people are not used to, or equipped for, the decadent non-stop way the city sucks in the unprepared. This is a city where there are no last calls, no time when a party can't be found. If you're not ready, it can swallow you into that dark place and never let you go.

For the local medic, it is a time of controlled chaos. It's kind of like being a bull rider, but instead of 8 seconds, your ride lasts 12 days.

This chaos is excepted as part of your right of passage, even looked forward too by those with a streak for debauchery.

In an epic clash of poor timing, Mardi Gras and the completion of my training as a Paramedic overlapped. This meant that all through the Mardi Gras season I would be working everyday as usual but every call would be scrutinized by a preceptor (a senior medic tasked with observing my techniques and judging my competence) during arguably the busiest time of the year.

My unit for this night shift would be composed of three people. My preceptor would be E.J., a skilled paramedic and normally the shift supervisor. Due to how busy we were, he got stuck on the truck with us. My other partner and fellow student on this shift would be Ray AKA 'Mad Dog'.

This combination was a strong high energy group and had the potential to be a lot of fun mixed with insanity.

The call was a typical Mardi Gras call. It was dispatched as two men not responsive. Possible overdose. They could be found on the ground outside the club 'Café Lafitte in Exile' on Bourbon St.

We pull up to the front doors of the bar into a sea of people. The bouncer standing at the club door just points with a bored expression to left of the door at two lumps of flesh on the ground. Hmmm, this could be interesting. They don't look so good.

We decide on the spot that we will grab a spine board, put one guy on it, and get him in the truck on the bench seat. That way, I can start working on him and then Ray and E.J. will go back and get the second guy with the stretcher.

We grab the first guy, get him in the truck and it's obvious that he is barely breathing. I mean like 2 or 3 times a minute barely.

My job at that point is to help him breath. The best way for me to do that (and make my preceptor write good things about me) is to intubate my patient. Intubation is the process of inserting a tube, via the mouth or nose, down into the trachea. It is then secured and a bag is attached to squeeze to push in air, assisting the patient in breathing.

Step 1: Open the airway......This guy has his jaws locked down tight. There is no getting his mouth open. The rest of his body is like a wet noodle, but his jaw is sealed.

Step 1.5: If you can't go in via the mouth then nasal (nose) intubation is next up to try. I am squatting down at his head. I have my tube in my right hand. I have my laryngoscope sitting next to his head (its no use if I can't get his mouth open) and I am cradling his head as I slide the tube into his right nostril.

Something way deep in his lizard brain does not like this tube sliding into his head because as soon as the tube made the gentle popping sound that signals it has entered his sinuses, his right hand moves with incredible speed and grabs me by the throat!

At the same time, E.J. and Mad Dog are loading the other patient in the truck. E.J. decided it's kind of crowded so he is going to go up front to drive, while we tend to the patients. Mad Dog sees me red faced trying to pry this guy's hand from my throat and thinks......well I'm not sure what he thinks. Whether he thought I was fucking around or what, but he starts laughing as he's closing the doors and getting in. At some point he realized that I wasn't playing. He could see that as I pulled the tube out of the patient's nose and was flogging him with it in an effort to get him to let me the hell go!

When looking to Ray for assistance, I know that there is only one response and that response will be very direct, no finesse, just straight up hammer versus nail and at the moment I didn't care I just wanted help.

Ray dives onto this guy's lap. He reaches out with one hand and grabs a large handful of crotch. He yells "MOTORBOAT!!" and starts to pull on the guys junk like the starter cord on a 60s Evinrude. I can't say for sure that this action loosened the grip on my neck since the world was starting to go black at the edges, but I was finally able to pry his hand free.

The very moment that his hand was free of my throat he went completely limp again. I take a huge breath and the sudden realization strikes me that we are not out of the woods yet.

It seems that the well-lubricated crowd had been watching this play by play through the windows and thought we were simply assaulting one of their fellow revelers. They responded by starting to rock the ambulance. It's amazing how much motion you can get in a unit with a hundred drunk people pushing. E.J., trapped in the front seat has called a 10-55 (officer needs assistance) on the radio and is trying to use the siren to ward off the worst of the mob.

The Calvary finally arrives in the form of our rescue truck and another ambulance and with their assistance we are able to creep out of the crowd.

Several hours later after I've had my throat X-rayed (just contused) and have gone and run more calls, I found myself back at Charity Hospital where we had left our patients earlier. The guy that had choked me out was sitting up in bed. He had no clue what had happened and was so apologetic that I thought he was going to cry. I wanted to be pissed at him, but it was really hard since the only thing he couldn't understand is why his testicals hurt so bad?

STREET FACE

One of the things besides medical skills that make the difference between an average medic and a really good medic (which I would like to think I am) are the intangibles. In my case (and in most great medics I know) it is the ability to not get ruffled. To not show your stress outwardly. I am known for telling my patients not to worry, that as long as I am laughing and smiling they will be fine. If things were really bad I'd be a lot more serious. This ability has been pushed, right to the limits, on several occasions and this story is about one of those times.

My partner and I were just clearing Charity Hospital and were the only unit not on a call. In a very urgent voice one of the other units came over the radio saying that a car had just struck his partner, a policeman, and a fireman. They were all on an accident scene they were working on Interstate 610.

We immediately took off toward the area they were in while dispatch updated us on the information of the call.

We arrived on scene to find that a drunk driver had run off the road and struck the back of the parked car that had previously been in an accident. Everyone was standing between the car and the ambulance. The policeman and fireman were up on their feet with minor injuries. My immediate focus was to the paramedic that was struck. Tony had been thrown over the concrete centerline divider landing in the opposing lanes. He was pretty shaken up and it appeared that he might have a fractured hip. This was a friend of mine. Someone that worked alongside of me, had been to my house and shared drinks and broken bread. This was no longer just a Patient, it was a friend, and focus would be a hard battle to fight.

We got Tony packaged up as with any accident victim and loaded him into the truck. I knew he understood what was about to happen but needed all the emotional support I could give. We were headed to Charity with him being considered a major trauma case.

I'm sitting on the bench looking down at Tony I'm prepping the first of two large bore IVs but trying to keep my banter up at the same time.

Tony's face is scared. I stop what I'm doing and look him in the eye with a smile on my face and channel all my will power into my next words.

"You're all good. This is standard precaution bullshit. You'll need to act sicker at the hospital if you want sympathy from the nurses."

Tony puts on a feeble smiles and relaxes some as I scramble to finish all my tasks. He knows I am a world class liar, and that I'd say anything to keep him calm but he lets my false words flow over him and for that moment denies his personal thoughts and allows me to assuage his fears.

I finish assessing my friends injuries, start my IVs, get him on oxygen, all while trying to hold his hand. I am not sure if holding his hand was helping him or me more.

We get to the hospital, the back doors open and he looks right up at me and says to me "Don't go far." with pleading eyes. I know I have become his anchor in this traumatic event. He needs me to help him keep the panic down. The only problem is the more I try and smile and stay confident my little voice is screaming and freaking out.

I go with him into the trauma room as they cut the remaining parts of his uniform away. A dozen hands are on him at once doing everything imaginable in an effort to classify his injuries. I turn his hand over to a nurse we both know. I make eye contact with her and I know she understands the situation and grasps his hand firmly. My respect for her has just climbed through the ceiling.

I walk out to the hall and find a scrub sink to wash up. Now that there is no one watching me the shakes start. My breathing is ragged and my hands shake uncontrollably. I know this is all the pent up adrenalin and fear from the call but it still rocks me to the core. I finally control my breathing. I rinse my face and take long slow meditative breaths.

Once I feel I am squared away I bury that fear again and put my street face back on so that I can see my friend and also face whatever else the City has to throw at me.

DEATH BY MISADVENTURE

Every medic, no matter how good he or she is (or thinks he is) had to be the new guy at some point. Probably several some points in his or her career. First days at a new service. First times as a team leader on calls, but the first that can be the hardest for all medics are your first days as an honest to God Paramedic. You no longer have the safety net of being a student and if you work for the City of New Orleans its time to be thrown to the wolves. It is considered a trial by fire where a new city Paramedic is placed in a truck. They are paired with one of the more aggressive paramedics. One that will push them and expect the very most from them.

Jenn was placed with me and my orders were to push her and see if she would break. She had done well and we were partners and friends as we neared the close of our two weeks together.

The call we received was odd from the beginning. It came from dispatch as an unknown Death in a French Quarter apartment. The address was a swanky condo type in an old world building.

We arrived and NOPD was already there which, for an unknown death, is not normal. Those guys have a response time measured with a calendar not a stop watch. My partner grabbed the cardiac monitor and I, the most important medical tool, the clipboard, and headed up the stairs.

As we entered the apartment it had more of the appearance of a domestic disturbance than a death. There was a 30ish guy standing in the middle of the room. He was very well dressed and crying in great sobs. The NOPD officer that was next to him with his handy dandy clipboard was taking down information between the sobs.

The Officer looks up and says "The bathroom."

Hmmmm....The plot thickens.

Jenn and I walked across the living area of the loft and turn into the large bathroom.

Lying on the floor on his side was a very naked, very handsome, very well built and very dead white guy in his late twenties or early thirties, but none of that was what struck me on first glance. It was that at first glance it appeared that he had at least 18 inches of penis laying across the floor.

Jenn turned in and got her first look. I can't say whether it was because of her newness as a paramedic, her normally loud vocal nature or her fascination with large member that made her respond as she did.

In a loud and throaty voice Jenn said "OH FUCKIN GAWD IS THAT HIS COCK!?!?"

From the other room, the man with the police officer let out an elevated wail.

On closer inspection it was not his penis but a humungous dildo that was in his ass and twisted between his legs and laid on the floor. Later follow up with the medical examiner revealed that it had been used on him vigorously until it had ruptured his colon leading to his death.

"Jenn, call it in to medical control."

Now for a woman who never seemed to hold her tongue she suddenly was struck mute. Shaking her head vigorously with her hands out in a warding off gesture I had finally found her weakness.....Talking about death by dildo.

"Fine I'll call it in." I got on the radio and called medical control so that I could get a declaration of death. The doctor I got on the radio is a great doc, a good guy, but his English......not so much.

"Doc I'm on scene with an approximately 30 year old white male. He is lying right lateral recumbent on the bathroom floor. He is pulseless, apneic and asystole in all three leads. He has rigor present. There is a large phallic object imbedded in his rectum."

"10-9?" (Please repeat)

"Doc he has a large phallic objected that's in his rectum."

"10-9?"

"Doc he has a giant dildo stuck in his ass!! Do you understand?"

Silence....lots and lots of Silence

"Doc you there?"

"Time of death 830am.......good bye."

~~DRIVE THRU BBQ~~

Summer holidays anywhere in the states are a great day to have fun, enjoy some grilling and maybe a few adult beverages, but New Orleans is not like anywhere else. Everything ends up being taken just one step to far.

I was working night shift as the Rescue Tech on Memorial Day. The street units were getting run hard but as rescue I had been very quiet.

The easy night was finally broken. The call finally came. It was a motor vehicle accident on Broad St. A truck had struck the concrete portion of a pumping station that protrudes into the street.

The street unit and I arrive at the same time. What we find is hard to believe. A 70s pick-up truck with a driver in the front and three BBQers in the back. Yes that's what you read. Three guys 0had been standing in the bed of the truck with a UFO charcoal grill loaded down with chicken taking their celebration on the road.

As we all walked toward the scene there were bodies, chicken pieces, and hot coals all sizzling on the street. The guys from the back of the truck were broken, braised and burnt as we tried collecting them for care.

The driver of the truck was not so lucky the impact had trapped him in the driver's seat when the dash rolled forward. We had to use the jaws to cut him free all the while trying to run IVs and dodge chunks of burning coal or sizzling chicken.

If you have ever heard someone talk about how an event can go sideways, this story explains what that means.

A LEGEND

I was told today that a man I've known for 25 years died today. I can't claim to have been a close friend, just an acquaintance to him and his daughter. We moved in and out of the same circles where his gravitational field was huge. As a young medic with a drive to learn all there is to know about trauma care Dr. Norman McSwain was a god. The pioneer of PHTLS and ATLS his programs literary are the books by which we medics live when it comes to trauma.

He was good about treating people like people. Some doctors seem aloof, but he never felt that way to me. His daughter worked alongside us for a time which I feel made us all seem closer to him. His parties and the George Dickel whiskey were things to remember.

The Louisiana Bureau of EMS posted the below list credited to Dr. Mcswain and I think it sums up his thoughts damn well.

McSwain's Rules of Patient Care

1. Death is your adversary and competitor, fight to win.

2. Treat the patient as if they were your mother, father or child.

3. Each minute has only 60 seconds. Do not waste any of them.

4. Assume nothing, trust no one, do it yourself.

5. Know anatomy cold.

6. Be technically quick.

7. Do not panic in the face of blood.

8. Work with physiology, not against it

9. Maintain energy production.

10. Know what to fix and what to leave alone.

11. Know when to run.

12. Paranoia prevents disasters.

a. The patient's disease is out to embarrass you.

b. The patient does not tell you the whole truth.

c. The most severe injury is under the unremoved clothes.

d. The infection is hidden by the dressing.

e. The patient has a problem that you do not know about.

13. Never talk a patient into or out of any operation.

14. The nurses' notes do not say what the nurse told you.

15. Do not procrastinate. Make a decision and carry it out.

16. Learn from your successes and from your failures.

17. Always question everything you do.

18. Don't whine, just get the job done.

Norman McSwain, MD, FACS

Great chest cutter, excellent teacher, damn good guy. I hope I can be remembered as well by so many.

DEEP FREEZE

Part of the love of being in EMS is that you never know what the next call is going to be. The wheel of fate spins and the next call arrives,

"Dispatch to 504?"

"Go ahead for 504."

"504 we have a signal 29 (death) on a ship currently traveling up the Mississippi."

"I'm sorry dispatch did you say on a moving ship?"

"Roger that. You need to proceed to Port Ship services. They have a crew boat that will take you to the ship. Our understanding is he died several days ago while at sea and they made notification when the river pilot came aboard."

"Um,......OK Dispatch."

We headed to the crew boat dock and got on the back deck. Off we went into the river. There we were lugging all our gear and I asked the deckhand on the boat what ship we were going to? He pointed to this rather large cargo ship moving up the river towards us. Wait, what? It's moving. How in holy hell are we going to get on that thing?

As we pulled alongside this moving mountain we saw the cargo net hanging down the side as an invitation to us. The ship was not going to stop for us, it really couldn't stop for us. At low speed it is nearly impossible to steer so they can't stop.

We grabbed our gear, strapped it to our backs and stepped to the edge of the crew boat. Now the trick to this, I was told by the deckhand as we stand there, is to jump and not miss. The moving crew boat was matching the speed with this ship and we jumped onto the hanging cargo net. As I clung for life on the cargo net I thought, I hope I don't have to do this in reverse to get off this damn thing.

We make it to the deck and are waived over by an Asian crew member that obviously doesn't speak English. He led us into the main areas of the ship. We were taken to the Galley where we were met by the First mate that spoke about twelve words of English which is why he was sent to communicate with us. He took us back through the kitchen to the deep freeze. There lying on the floor is a frozen dead guy.....our patient.

This guy had been dead for days. Hell, he had been frozen solid for days. He was lying next to a stack of fish fillets. I am no doctor but I don't think they needed anything from me.

We did the paperwork. We welcomed the dead guy to America and pronounced him officially dead as his welcoming gift. Once it was all done the crew invited us to stay for lunch...........The menu for the meal included fish.......We declined.

BRIGHT FIELD

It was a beautiful Saturday afternoon, at the peak of the Christmas shopping season in 1996 when a 735-foot bulk cargo ship called the M/V Bright Field lost engine power and collided with the River Walk shopping center, Hilton hotel, and the Pier condominiums.

The scared frightened people that were there fled in all directions leaving their belongings in place. At the Daiquiri store right where the impact happened a drink sat with ice still in it and a pipe with smoke still drifting serenely from its bowl.

The jewelry store looked perfectly intact except that the entire rear wall was gone and had fallen into the river.

As rooms in the hotel were searched, NOFD team members would check the room doors for heat (in case of fire) and then would pop the lock and search the rooms. One room that the door was popped on opened on absolutely nothing on the other side, no room at all, just open space over the Mississippi River.

At one point looking down in the river the rescuers saw what they believed to be a person that has fallen in. On closer inspection it was merely mannequins.

It was one of the surrealist scenes I have ever been on, made even more so by the fact that such a tragic event had, thankfully, no fatalities and only 66 injuries none of them severe.

~~ARE YOU A COP~~ ~~~~~~~~~~~~~~~~~~~~~~~~~~~~~~~~~~

Mardi Gras is so much fun if you're a people watcher, and as a medic there are times when you can stand back, away from the crowds and observe. During the parade season, units are strategically placed around the city to handle the increased calls in those areas. My favorite place to be staged was on the corner of Bourbon St. and Toulouse St. We would park the truck facing away from Bourbon, open the back doors and drag a barricade behind the truck and we had a ready-made med area. This allowed us to watch all the craziness while keeping the unwashed hoard at an acceptable distance.

It's the Saturday before Fat Tuesday and we are on our station. My partner, Scott and I have been here since 8am and things have been steady but we know the flood of humanity will start soon. It's only 3pm and the crowds are growing.

We are standing at our barricade looking like ranch hands leaning on the rail with one foot on the bottom bar just watching the crowd.

A fairly pretty, scantily clothed, and completely drunk girl in her 30s, with a neck full of beads saunters up to our barricade. She looks at me and with a slur of syllables she says "Are you a cop?" I respond "Nope." and she proceeds to flash her titties at me.

My partner is all of 18 inches away from me. He is dead silent through this entire exchange. He has that disapproving look on his face (once you get to know him you realize that's just the way he looks).

The girl slides down the barricade to Scott and scrutinizes him closely. She asks the same question. "Are you a cop?" My partner is silent and stone faced.

She seems amused instead of angry by his silence and steps closer.

She asks again "Are you a Cop?" but without waiting for an answer she shoots her hand between the bars of the barricade and fondles him with vigor. Scott's look of surprise will be forever in my mind.

The girl lets go of his privates, steps back and says "Well you don't feel like a cop." and walks back into the crowd leaving him slack jawed and confused with me laughing uncontrollably.

~~DIRECTIONS~~

Everyone knows that one of the worst things in the world to have is a bored teenager. A bored medic is not too far behind in this regard. Medics will go to great lengths to entertain themselves on those rare slow shifts.

A long standing Mardi Gras tradition that EMS has adopted from the Police Department is the giving of directions to tourists.

You're stationed at a location watching the people pass you by, maybe a little envious of them drinking and having fun. People routinely come up and ask for directions. Where is Brennan's Restaurant? Where can I pee? How do I get to Mardi Gras? (No shit they actually ask that.)

At the begin of the Mardi Gras season you are chipper and helpful giving detailed directions with a smile. Knowing it's the right thing to do and it helps pass the time. As the days wear on and the volume of hours and number of calls begin to take a toll, you stop giving helpful friendly directions; at some point you stop giving clipped short directions. Finally you give no directions looking at the people as if they have grown a third eye.

It's about this time you dawn your secret sarcastic identity. Pulling out that non-official name tag reserved for just this time of year. It reads Mr. DILLIGAF. What pray tell is so special about this name tag? First it's not your name. When a complaint gets made later they may describe you but they won't get your name right. More importantly, it's a secret code to the other members of your tribe. The cops, Fireman, and medics from around the country. They will see this name tag and know you are not to be trusted with factual information.

Like all government type jobs acronyms are a major part of your life, so much so that you even have them for your mischief. You are announcing to the world:

Mister **D**o **I** **L**ook **L**ike **I** **G**ive **A** **F**uck?

Now safe within the protective shell of your disguise you are free to wreak havoc.

Mr. Farmers tan from Middle America asks "Where is Café Du Monde?" You say "Two blocks up, take a right."

Ms. I'm away from home for the first time asks "How do I find a taxi?" You say "Two blocks up, take a right."

A gaggle of young men ask "where are the best strippers at?" You say "Two blocks up, take a left." This will send them to the police station as an extra insult.

Year after year this is the directions you give and they never seem to come back to you and say you were wrong……..

I have always wondered if there was a dead end alley two blocks up on the right that has a heard of people standing in it staring at the walls like lost sheep.

CORDITE AND MAHJONG

On one of my visits to San Francisco I rode shotgun with my friend Sebastian, who was a Captain at the time with the City EMS service. I quickly came to realize an age old truth. Big cities are the same on the large scale, but different on the small scale.

The calls of injuries and illnesses were very similar to what we saw in New Orleans, but the subtlety of the personalities and culture were unique.

A unit was dispatched to an alley in China Town for a shooting. It was close to midnight at the time and we, just so happened, were less than a block away.

We turned into the alley to locate our patient. Windows were down listening and looking for clues. The alley was completely deserted but you could smell the heavy pungent odor of Cordite where weapons had been fired just moments ago. The hairs on my neck were standing up knowing the gunman had been missed by mere seconds.

As we eased our way out the alley the only sound on the air was the sounds of Mahjong tiles being shaken somewhere in the buildings getting ready for the next round of betting in the gambling parlor.

SPIDER BITE

The only thing worse than a call at 2am is a bullshit call at 2am. My partner this night was Robin. She and I had a lot in common we both had very little tolerance for bullshit and we liked the same type of women, so we made excellent partners.

Static....."6215, 6215, Report of a possible broken arm." The address was in the Desire housing projects just a ½ mile from where we were. We grumbled, moaned, and got on the road.

As we pulled into the court yard for our address a guy of about 30 or so came walking out of the building right up to our unit.

"Ya'll here for the broken arm?" He said.

"Yea, where are they at?" I asked.

"It's me, I'm the one who called." Our now patient advised.

Well we got pissed and quick. He looked fine and was calling an ambulance. I started to read him the riot act and he started to apologize.

He said he was sorry and that he was embarrassed to tell the person on the phone what was wrong. I looked over to Robin and elevated my eyebrows. She just shrugged.

"Tell us what's going on." I said in an attempted calm voice.

"Well you see lass night I wenn to da club down da street. It was abouts fo in the moaning when I leffs and I was tired, so I's cut across the field wit da high grass. I stopped by the ole wall 'cause I had to piss an when I had it out I tink somin bite me."

"On your Penis?" I asked for clarification

"well yea, but I was tired so I wenn to bed. I wokes up dis morning an got up to piss an it was swole but it didn't hurt much so's I wenn back to bed. I got up this evenin an it was still pretty swole, but I had erens to run. I jus woke up a lil while ago an its still swole bad so I thoughts I better let somun look at it."

My partner immediately whispers "you look at it, it's not my area of experience"

I respond "Not exactly mine either!"

We settle it with the ultimate level of fairness and democracy. Rock, Paper Scissors.

I lose...............

Alright come on my friend get in the back of this truck and let's figure this out.

I get in the back with him. I'm sitting on the bench seat and he is standing / crouching in the back.

"Let's see it." I said in a voice devoid of any enthusiasm.

He unhooks and lowers his pants. The last 3 or 4 inches of his penis are grossly deformed. The end is swollen making it look like the head on a sledge hammer in its disfigurement. It's discolored and oozing an unknown fluid.

He grabs it by the shaft and informs me, as he vigorously shakes it, that "See it done even hurt that bad!!"

"Whoooaa my friend why don't you put that anaconda away and we will take you to the hospital."

PRANKS

In any tight knit group a level of familiarization happens that leads to less than professional pranks on each other. Here are a few of the evil items of mischief and mayhem I have either given or received.

The sardine can:

New Orleans is hot, so placing an open can of sardines under other the trucks seat of another unit and letting it bake in the heat is childish but damn funny.

Baby powder vents:

Did I mention New Orleans was hot? When another crew is away from their truck you turn off the batteries so nothing works (There's a switch next to the driver's seat). You then turn the air conditioning all the way up. You spray baby powder into the vents. When they come back and start the truck a giant cloud greets them.

The nasal cannula:

One tool used regularly on the ambulance is called a nasal cannula. It is a clear plastic tube about 5 foot long. One end hooks to the oxygen bottle the other has two little prongs that go in your nose to supply you with more oxygen. This tool has other evil options though. If you wedge the nasal prongs between the seat and the seat back of your partners spot so that they just extended to where he or she would be sitting. Then run the length of tubing out of sight behind the chairs and to the door side of your seat. You can then load up a 50cc or larger syringe with warm water and magically it fits on the end of the nasal cannula.

Now as you drive down the street you act as casual as possible and slowly squeeze the syringe. You get one of two responses. The first is instant freak out, where they jump up and start cursing. The second is more subtle and so much more rewarding. As you squeeze out the water you're watching them and you see them squirm. They are not sure if they just peed themselves so they sit silent and embarrassed. That's when you give them a little more...lol...and suddenly they are looking for a place to stop.

Nitro Paste:

How to take a valued cardiac medicine and make a toy out of it. Medics and mad scientists have a lot in common, foremost is that they will use their evil genius to entertain themselves. Nitro paste is designed to dilate your blood vessels and lower your blood pressure. It is used in different cardiac cases.

When medics use it for sport it can be dangerous. The most common of all the ways it is used is under the door handles of other people's trucks. You smear a glob (while wearing gloves) under the door handle where it can't be seen. When the person comes out the reach up they get a good handful and within seconds they get a profound headache and feel faint. Yes it is childish. Yes it is dangerous. Yes I have done it many times.

Vaseline on wipers:

I don't need to explain how evil this can be, do I? Especially in a city where rain is pretty common.

CATS

There are certain calls that stay with you as long as you live. These can be funny, sad, or have some other deep impact on you. Some tap into a visceral fear that you can't shake no matter how hard you try.

We were called to an apartment in an area known for being low rent, fixed income folks. We were on a health and welfare check. That's when a family member from out of down hasn't heard from their loved one in a while and is concerned enough to dial 9-1-1. We would go out in the ambulance and check on them. Most times it was simply communication break down since this was in the pre-cellphone era and most of these people were older and not likely to have pagers. This gentleman hadn't been heard from in about a week.

As soon as we got to the door, we knew this was not a friendly check. It was summer, this place obviously didn't have air conditioning and we were hit with the smell of a dead body.

We tracked down the land lord and got the key to the door. When the door opened the heat and smell made a physical impact like a slap to the face. It was the putrid smell of decay but it was overlaid with other smells, namely ammonia.

Our first steps in showed a house filled with cats. There were easily a dozen in the main room shewing cats as we went. We made our way across the apartment's entry room to finish our search. We searched the house and when we got to the bathroom we found the gentleman we were looking for. He was naked, on his knees, face down in the toilet. He had obviously had a major Gastrointestinal bleed. There was dried coffee ground like blood everywhere in the room. I can only assume that he never had the strength to get to the phone to call for help. He died kneeling on the bathroom floor surrounded by his cats........at least a week ago.

As we are standing there I am stunned into immobility by movement, movement below him. Then I see it. A cats head coming out of the man. The cat climbed completely out of a hole through the rectum area that it (and the others I surmise) had chewed as they used their owner as sustenance over the past week.

I freaked. I have to say that I did not walk out......I ran. I've never liked cats since that day and damn sure won't let them lick my face.......

SWEET METER

The wee hours of the morning, near the end of your shift, is always the hardest time to keep awake and focused. If you have a small thing like diabetes, it can cause even more issues.

On one of these tough early mornings, I was cleaning out my truck on the ramp at charity, when dispatch gave a call to the truck that was parked on the street in front of the E.R. The medics were both in the front seats just napping, killing the end of the shift. I saw the medic in the passenger seat tap the driver, who then set up, pulled the vehicle in drive, and hit the gas. They made it down the block and made the right turn at the end..............

That's when things started to go wrong. The driver although awake was not really with it. He was the diabetic. His blood glucose was low, so he was not really oriented. He had enough focus to get the vehicle in drive hit the gas and the last command was turn right.

So as my unit left the hospital, just seconds behind them, we found that their unit had made the right turn and just kept turning. It had turned up over a parking meter and was just spinning its wheels. Our sugar depleted friend in the driver's seat was locked in a feed-back loop. His foot was on the throttle one hand on the wheel and one on the gear shifter.

This is where the real problems start. See the fact that he drove the truck up on the grass is no big deal. The problem is he hit the meter. The meter is the City of New Orleans' property. If the meter is reported hit, our friend will need a police report and someone may cause him grief that he was out of it. If the meter went away, well, no harm, no foul.

My partner and I decided to help out and make the meter disappear. We got the truck off of it and put it in our unit on the stretcher. We then reported to dispatch that there was an issue.

What we didn't expect was Dispatch giving us the first units call.....crap.....not thinking enough steps ahead.

It's an O B call (pregnant women). Dispatch's description makes us think it won't require transport. We are idiots, so we head to the call and leave the meter on the stretcher.

We get to the call address and the girl is standing on the front porch with a suitcase......sigh.

OK, partner goes to the girl. I open the back of the truck, grab the meter, and sneak out the side door of the unit. This is done as he loads the patient into the back. It's the keystone medics. I stow the meter in the side cabinet, head to the driver's seat and off we go with the patient.

After delivering the girl we are now running out of time to our shift. It's almost time to turn in the truck and at the moment that would be bad. There is just enough time to run to the river.

We get to the Mississippi river dock and with little fanfare (but we did look to make sure we weren't observed). We send the parking meter to a watery grave. When I have told this story in the past I am always asked; "Why didn't you keep it?" The answer is easy. If we kept it that would be theft. If anyone ever asks, we know right where the meter is and we were keeping it safe.

MAW FRAN

My Great Grandmother was an ornery old bird. She lived in New Orleans when I was working as a paramedic for the city. She was in her 90's and lived alone. She fancied dialing 9-1-1 and asking for an ambulance and me, by name! She would say she needed an ambulance but wanted me to come pick her up.

This particular day she called and said she was short of breath to send me to get her. My partner and I started in that direction but as fate would have it, our truck broke down as soon as we started rolling. The day shift Supervisor, Wayne, was good enough to say he would go there and assess her condition and stay with her until we could get there.

We swapped from our broken truck to a working truck and headed that way. Wayne told us he was there and sitting with her and would meet us at the door.

When we arrived at her house Wayne meets us and begins to say what a nice old lady my Grand-maw is. I lean back and look at the house numbers. When I do he asks me why. I tell him I wasn't sure he went to the right address because that didn't sound like my Great Grandmother. He laughs at me as we head in the house. I am pretty sure he thought I was joking.

Maw Fran is sitting in her chair and I can tell she has a cold, so I ask what she wants us to do and if she thinks she needs to go to the hospital. Of course she does. I tell her to get up and walk to the stretcher. She glances furtively at Wayne and my partner and says, "I can't get up." I tell her she needs to get up and walk out to the stretcher because I know she can walk and if she wants a ride she better start helping us.

Wayne is looking at me as if I have a third eye. He says you don't have to be rude to your Grandma like that. Before I can comment to him Maw Fran says to the room "See how nice he is, even for a darkie."

Well I am mortified by this. Wayne's jaw is wide open at first, but then he just laughs it off. I apologize for her and with his hands buried in his pockets he says "It's alright Bo, it ain't your fault let's get her in the truck."

We get her loaded into the truck and Wayne is standing at the back doors as I get her situated. She takes that moment to cough up a big loogey and spit it right on the ambulance floor. I get very irate over this and start giving her all kinds of hell. Wayne of course tells me that I shouldn't speak to her that way. Wayne is a good southern man and very respectful of the elderly. He is of course right but at the moment I was fairly annoyed.

Before Wayne or I could say anything else Maw Fran chimed in "You should listen to him. He's pretty smart, for a negro."

Oh, holy mother of misspoken words, did she really just say that? I look over at Wayne's face and yep, from his expression, she most certainly did say it. He looks at me and says "You're on your own with this one my Brother." And closes the rear doors.

MECHANICAL DIFFICULTY

Not everything that happens that is crazy on a call is due to the patient or the medic. The main supporting cast is the Ambulance, our home and office for our 12 hour shift.

At one point in my career I worked for a local Sheriff's Office that had a Rescue/ EMS Division. The importance of this is that all the Police cars and Ambulances got serviced by the jail's inmates. It was cheap but I wouldn't call it effective.

My partner Andre was driving our van ambulance while I was in the back with a nice older lady that had been having chest pain. We are proceeding down the road when Andre calls to me. "Hey can you stick your head up here?"

I stick my head through to the front of the unit. "What's up?"

He just points out the passenger window. I look in that direction and see the strangest thing ever. The front tire is a good three feet outside of the wheel well and as Murphy's law will have it we are just coming into a left handed curve in the road.

As calmly as I can, I tell my patient that there may be a bit of a bump. I wedge myself in the doorway between the cab and the patient compartment as I watch the wheel and the whole spindle roll away from the truck. Andre is trying to steer to keep the truck balanced on three wheels but the road continues to turn to the left.

We finally reach the tipping point and the unit heaves over onto the bumper and passenger front panel. There is a loud screeching and grinding as we come to a stop. The truck is tilted all crazy. The ass of the truck is elevated. My patient is rattled. This is becoming a difficult day.

There was insult to be added to our injury. We called for another ambulance to help our patient finally get to the hospital and learned that the stretcher was never designed to be removed when canted and elevated!

So the final quiz is how many medics must stand on the rear bumper of a unit to get it level enough to remove granny chest pains from the rear?.......

"WE KNOW YOU'RE ALRIGHT…"

In the days following hurricane Katrina communication from inside the city with anyone in the outside world was extremely limited and very difficult. This was compounded by my lack of understanding regarding text messaging.

The cell phone lines were obviously inundated with people trying to get calls in and out. The local towers were either down or damaged making normal communication all but impossible.

I received my first text message ever, in the wee hours of the morning. Our way of attempting communication was to wait until after midnight, go up to the highest point on the Mississippi River Bridge, and try and get cell service from the neighboring area's cell towers. One of the first nights I attempted this my phone made a sound I hadn't heard before and with some investigation found the text message.

The text was from friends of my wife and I. They knew we both had stayed in the city to work. It read "We know you're alright, how is Rose?" I took this to mean that they had confidence in my abilities to take care of myself and was concerned for my wife because she was pregnant for our son at the time. I know, I'm modest aren't I?

As the days passed I continued to receive text messages from friends all over the United States. They all expressed the same message. We know your all right and some other question or thought. There was little I could do to figure this small mystery out plus I had a lot of other things on my mind at the time.

A little more than a week after the storm I was able to take my wife north of New Orleans to family, before I returned to my duties I obviously took the opportunity for a hot shower, food, and clean clothes. While waiting for my clothes, I remember being mesmerized by the video on the major news channels. Much of what was playing I was told was repeated over and over from the first days after landfall.

As I am watching the talking heads and the endless news reel I saw....well I saw ME. A video of me in uniform loading a wounded Police Officer in the back of an Ambulance. I had to think, when the hell was this? I don't recall the camera. I asked family if they had seen this and they said that they saw me load that patient about once an hour for the last week. Everyone knew I was okay, because I was making the national news play by play and I didn't even know it.

AFRICAN FRIEND

As a medic I have had the great pleasure to travel all over the world. I have taught in other countries. I have acted as a Remote Medical Specialist for private groups and corporations. This has allowed me to have what appears on the surface a glamorous career.

Well looks can be deceiving. I was a Remote medical specialist on an oil platform off the coast of Africa near the Congo River basin. I had just arrived and hadn't even gotten settled into my clinic when one of the locals that was stationed on the rig came in to see me. His English was not bad as he introduced himself and shook my hand.

He asked me "We friends?" I said sure I can always use friends. He next said "You check me?" Well I am the medic and said sure I'll check you what's wrong? I'm thinking to myself he needs his blood pressure checked or has some old injury he needs me to inspect. I was wrong!

As soon as I said sure I'll check you, he turned around pulled his pants down, bent over at the waste and spread the cheeks of his ass.

WHOOOOAAA.......

It seems that my new friend had hemorrhoids and wanted them checked out. As important as friendships are I feel that I was going to be a bit shy making new local friends.

OXYGEN

Some of the things you see as a medic are shocking, confusing or just downright bizarre. One such thing that always troubled me was suicides. Understanding why someone would take their own life is very difficult for me to understand, much less understand why they choose the methods that they do to commit this act. I guess it's good that I don't understand, but it doesn't stop me from wondering.

It's an early morning and we are called to a home of an elderly lady that lives alone. Her concerned neighbor always drinks coffee with her in the morning and no one was answering the door.

The neighbor tells us that her friend is confined to a wheelchair and is on oxygen. She has terminal lung cancer and is in her 70s.

We finally are able to open a door and go inside and what we find is, at first, extremely confusing. This sick elderly lady was sitting in her wheelchair. 38 revolver in her lap and the entire top of her head from her nose on up is blown off. The ceiling and walls are a Jackson Pollock piece. What in the hell happened here?

As we investigate we find her Oxygen bottle mounted to her wheel chair and about two foot of hose still connected to it. The hose appears burned on the end.

Our conclusion goes something like this. Our terminal patient decided she was going to end her life before the lung cancer took any further toll on her. She got her .38 revolver and steadied herself for the grim task.

We believe that she placed the pistol in her mouth and then in a last attempt to fortify her nerve took a deep breath through her nose and held it. That deep breath was pure oxygen from nasal cannula and filled her sinuses.

When she pulled the trigger it caused her sinuses to act as a combustion chamber igniting the oxygen and causing complete devastation to her head.

~~TROOPER'S HAT~~

The call was as simple as it was silly. A reviler at a downtown Mardi Gras parade had been imbibing a bit much and decided to climb the barricades that line the parade route. When he got on the top of the 4 foot barricade he fell, ass over tea kettle onto the street, landing on his head.

Law Enforcement from New Orleans and Louisiana State Police, hold the street area inside the barricades and called us to treat our wayward partier. We approached from the side street and the crowd was easily 8 to 10 people deep. We waded through the crowd with our stretcher and was let through the barricade to the street.

Our patient was a little hurt and a lot of drunk. We needed to secure him to a spine board as our protocol required but he was having none of it. We have an audience of thousands watching so we try and GENTLY secure this guy down.

One of the State troopers walked over. He was tall and his uniform was perfect and pressed and, of course, he had on his ever present Smokey the Bear hat. He reached down to assist us. Our patient took that moment to get rowdy and swung his arm catching the Trooper on the brim of his hat. The hat launched straight up and went tumbling through the air. The crowd let out a combined eeeeewwwwww!! The Trooper having momentarily lost his composure punched my patient in the face with three rapid jabs. He then went in search of his hat.

Our patient being momentarily stunned was easy to secure to the spine board and get onto the stretcher. We began to make our way back through the crowd and a strange thing happened. The crowd that had obviously sided with the Trooper in the altercation, began to reach out of the throng of people and pummel our patient as we worked our way out of the crowd. They then let out a cheer as we loaded him in the ambulance to take him away. The crowd is fickle and you never know where their loyalties will be.

~~DEFIBRILLATOR DISTRESS~~

One of the many skills a Paramedic uses in his arsenal is the defibrillator. In very crude terms this machine is designed to send lots of electrical current through the human body, specifically the heart, in an attempt to reset it. Let me rephrase that, it's used on a person with no heartbeat. Technically it's used on a person that is dead. When not used on a dead person problems begin to arise.

In what seems to be a completely unrelated topic, New Orleans has a lot of great history and architecture. One place where the two come together is the shotgun house. This house as its name sake suggests is long and narrow. The rooms line up one behind the other. Calls in these can be tricky. Cardiac arrests can be a nightmare.

I was working a cardiac arrest in the kitchen of a shotgun house. This little bitty room and very large patient didn't leave a lot of space to work in. I had attached the cardiac monitor to him and was trying to get in a good position to work. Our patient had collapsed in front of the refrigerator and was sprawled to both sides. I was wedged against the handle side preparing to administer a shock.

Now normal procedure is to call "Clear", everyone has seen this done on TV. What it is meant to do is alert all the other (live) people in the room to make sure you are not in contact with the patient since they are about to have lots of electricity pushed through them.

I press the paddles down on the patient's chest and press the button delivering 300 joules of electricity into the patient, but it didn't stop there. It seems that his right arm which was blocked from my line of sight was touching the hinge side of the refrigerator and being a total surprise to me, my right foot was in contact with the handle side of the fridge.

It was a shock, pun intended, to me, when the electricity went into the patient, from him to the fridge, then out the fridge into me. It knocked me over, fried the fridge and tripped the breaker in the house. Now I had the twitches, on the floor in the dark, trying to find the patient. It was a hair raising ordeal.

PETE'S FISH FRY

One thing that medics are is nosey. We can't help it, part of our makeup is solving problems, and it's what makes us good medics. So as a group we all wish we had the most interesting calls and when we don't, we want to know what's happening on them and get the blow by blow.

One of our fellow night shift units were dispatched to a shooting at Pete's Fish Fry, a notorious location known for large crowds and occasional gunfire. Since we weren't given the interesting call, we would listen in on it.

The best way to snoop on this was to wait until you heard the unit arrive on scene. Once they were there either you or your partner would change your radio to the medical control channel. This channel was a direct link to the doctors at Charity hospital. It allowed the units to call in reports and request medical orders.

So, all these other medics are sulking in the dark pissed they didn't get the interesting fast paced call. Acting like peeping Tom's (listening Tom's?) waiting to hear the report from the scene.

"Paramedic Unit to Med Control."

"This is med control, go ahead."

"Doc, we are on scene with an approximately 25 year old male. He has a gunshot wound to his head. Appears to be a large caliber entry wound to the face below the left eye. He has a reciprocal exit wound posterior head which is gaping with gray matter exposed. Patient is pulseless, apneic, EKG shows asystole in all three leads. I'm requesting Do Not Resuscitate order (DNR)."

"Is he still warm?"

"Yes Doc, he is still warm, he has been down approximately 10 minutes."

"Have you begun CPR?"

"Doc let me repeat. He has a large entry and an extremely large exit wound in his head with a large quantity of gray matter removed."

"What are you trying to tell me?"

"Doc, I'm looking through the hole in his head and can read the song on the jukebox!!"

"DNR granted."

~~GRANDMA~~

One of the things you think about when you become a medic is your family. You think about how your newly acquired skills could be used to help your family in case of emergency. The thought is a noble one, picturing yourself as you ride in on a white horse. The reality is far different.

I was working night shift, which had always been my preference. I was living in a converted garage apartment behind my Grandparents' home. I was used to being awoken by my Grandfather as he cut the grass under my window or did some other outside, daytime activity. Today was a bit different.

I was shaken awake by my Grandpa. This was strange because normally he would never have come into my apartment without knocking. I opened my eyes and he looked worried bordering on scared. He said something was wrong with my Grandma.

I jumped out of bed and followed my Grandfather to his house grabbing my jump bag from my car on the way. My Grandmother was lying on the sofa, she was very pale and sweating, in short she looked bad.

I tell Grandpa to dial 911 and get a unit rolling. I check her pressure and its LOW....very low...crap, shit, damn-it. I have nothing but a BP cuff and a stethoscope. I am at a near state of panic having none of the tools of the trade, outside of my wits. Having just woken up they are pretty dull.

The unit gets there quick for them but what felt like a lifetime to me. The medics are co-workers of mine and are fantastic in helping me get my Grandmother loaded in the unit and begin treatment.

I hold her hand as we race to the hospital. I try my best to show a strong face and not let her see any of my scared feelings on top of her own. I realize as we are getting to the hospital, I was so freaked that I'm in the ambulance wearing just boxers and a t-shirt.

Between my patient report to the ER and my entrance in a state of undress the staff understood the seriousness of the problem and rushes to help. I am so grateful to have others there to bear the load of her care but the other side of it is I don't have anything to concentrate on but my fears for my Grandmother.....

I knew she would be okay when the nurses started to make fun of my fashion choices. I never thought embarrassment would be such a relief.

~~NASAL DOUCHE~~

Learning is part of life. We must constantly learn to move forward in life. Being a medic is no different but when you're brand new it seems like you know nothing and everything is crushing down on you as you try to stay on top of it all.

As EMT students, everything is new and foreign and in our first visit to the hallowed halls of Charity Hospital we are in awe. Everyone moved so fast, they tell us things and we stare like lemmings. My friend and I are put in a pod in the ER. This is an area of 4 beds. We are told to take vital signs on all four patients for practice. Okay, I think we can do that.

As we approach the bed side my partner Rob bumps the wall and knocks the oxygen line with a humidifier off the wall attachment and it falls to the floor. Oh crap, Rob, pick it up before someone sees it.

This humidifier is attached to our patient's nasal cannula. What it does is allows the dry oxygen to pass through water then bubble out of the water to be easier for the patient to tolerate.

Rob picked up the humidifier and looks at it.........hmmmmm how was this mounted to the wall? We both look around and no one else in the quad has one. Rob's guess is with the bottle up like an IV bag......That was the wrong answer.

The humidifier bottle goes down so the air can pass in then out of the liquid. Rob's solution caused the fluid to run down the line and shoot with vigor directly into both of the nice old lady's nostrils. The patient started thrashing about as she had her sinuses cleaned. We both froze as our feeble minds attempted to process the disaster. We finally get the thing back off the wall and out of the poor ladies nose

All Rob says as we are hauling ass out of the room is that there is no charge for that particular service. That nice lady said some of the most vulgar things toward us as we left.

~~BULLSHIT~~ AS TOLD BY M. HARRISON

This is the story I tell people (from our time together). Now you know I am Irish so I don't let the truth get in the way of a good story. I tell everyone you were a door gunner on a Huey flying missions in Central America taking rounds in your bird. Well remember Jack Stephens is the Sheriff at the time. We are in our monthly battle for funding from the Police Jury, the news stations are hanging on every move. After all, this is St. Bernard, the Parish that historically is closed to the media.

The Police Jury meeting goes on and on, we are there in uniform when the meeting adjourns. Once again we were afforded temporary funding. Everyone is frustrated. You have that look on your face, to say you were pissed is an understatement. All the News cameras are filming. One of them asks you what you thought. You looked at them and said. "I was a door gunner in combat and I much rather be shot at than have to deal with politics." The news man asked why? You said. "Bullets I can get out the way of. Politics, like Bullshit, covers everything."

The cameraman and News man started laughing their asses off. That made everything crystal clear. The News media wished they could put that on the air. It was great. The Sheriff pissed himself laughing. Then he was sure this EMS is worth fighting for. The Police Jury did not have a leg to stand on.

A LOVER'S SCORN

Anger and alcohol are combinations that we see all too often. The results, as these two elements clash, are some of the worst of humanity.

The call was for multiple patients, cut by a knife. As we arrive we see that it's in a rundown neighborhood of houses that have been divided up into multiple apartments.

I head down the dark alley that lead to the back steps and the apartment entrance we're looking for. I find the first victim sprawled at the bottom of the stairs. He is laying propped against the final steps of the landing in a lake of his own blood. He has the unmistakable look that a death brings. A mix of inanimate object mixed with a sense of wrongness. He is white, not just Caucasian, his skin is alabaster. It seems every drop of blood has left his body. He is shirtless and I can clearly see a stab wound on the left side of his chest between the fourth and fifth rib. I look closer with my flashlight and can actually see into his chest cavity.

There is nothing I can do hear. I leave him and head up the stairs. At the landing between the 1st and 2nd floor I clearly see where he met his end. The spray of blood on the wall and the first expulsion of his blood litter the landing along with the smears where he fell down the stairs to his position at the base of the landing. It is all clearly visible.

I walk into the apartment on the second floor and am met with several sites that are overwhelming in their oddity and severity. There is a man in his thirties standing naked in the center of the room. He has a vacant look in his eyes that is combined with that of horror, pain and fear in his expression. He is holding his right arm out away from his body, as if it has offended him. My first thought is why is a naked man wearing a long glove? It's not a glove. It's a de-gloving injury! He has been cut completely around his forearm and the skin has slid down like a ladies formal glove. I can now see the exposed muscle and sinew exposed as if in an anatomy lesson.

On the floor, in the corner of the room is a young female. She is naked and laying on her right side. She would be quite beautiful, if she wasn't scooping up her intestines off the floor and trying to stuff them back in her open abdomen. She has been cut completely across her belly in an arching wound like a giant smirk. The more she struggles to return her guts to her body the more horrific the scene appears.

We treat the patients that need treating, transporting them to the hospital for care. We return to the scene to complete the paperwork on the patient that was beyond our ability and scope of care. The police tell us the story that led to this bizarre scene.

Our female victim was drinking at a local watering hole having just separated from her steady lover. Our slasher, as it turns out, was that lover, and had decided to come to the same bar following her.

As one can imagine she was not pleased that he was following her. He was power drinking and giving her a hard time. She had a fairly unorthodox idea on how she planned to rub the separation in on our spurned lover. She went up to two men that were drinking together at the bar and invited them to go back to her apartment with her.

Our slasher stewed at the bar for a bit, letting the anger and frustration of his dismissal eat at him. In a reckless, alcohol fueled moment of rage he grabbed the huge bar knife, used to cut up lemons, and walked out. He hailed a cab and headed for his former lover's house. Upon getting there, he told the cabbie to wait. The cabbie stayed until he heard the screams then hauled ass and dialed 9-1-1.

As our killer headed up to the apartment. He must have announced his presence because lover #1 met him on the landing of the steps and was immediately stabbed to death. When he pushed his way into the apartment lover #2 stuck out his arm in a stop motion and had the flesh cut from his arm.

Our killer confronted his ex and she obviously did not grasp the gravity of the situation because she yelled and screamed at him. His response was to swing his knife in an arcing slash across her belly by luck or skill, the knife cut just deep enough to let her intestines tumble out.

He then walked out of the apartment and finding his cab gone, just walked up the street. He was picked up a few blocks away carrying the murder weapon, while covered in all three of his victim's blood.

SECOND GUESSES

One of the traits we think of when thinking of a paramedic is of someone that makes a decision in a split second, then is firm in that decision without any doubts. The reality is sometimes not that easy as we second guess calls over days, weeks even years. The ability to make these split second decisions is a must so also is the human side of living with the decisions we make.

It was a domestic dispute. Boyfriend and girlfriend both in their thirties, both fairly angry and hostile. She had been drinking and they were at his house. We were on the scene because of her being under the influence. The sheriff's Office, who we also worked for, was just trying to cover their collective asses.

She was threatening to hurt him for some indiscretion that has faded from my memory over time. He was very stoic and just wanted her out of his house. All in all not that uncommon of a situation.

It was decided to give her a ride to her house. We were to give her that ride for unknown reasons. As we headed to her place she was still very angry and made it clear that she was going to 'show' him. We dropped her off, even went so far as to walk her inside as I recall. She was immediately forgotten as we went on to our next call.

Several hours later we were stopped for lunch, I remember it very clearly. We were sitting at the diner counter. I was eating chicken parmesan with red gravy and spaghetti. The radio crackled and dispatch called us and another unit advising of a possible suicide. The address she gave was the girl's we had dropped off earlier. Thoughts run through your mind. This can't be true. I just talked to her. We of course raced to the scene.

She had a pistol at her house and had shot herself in the head. I argue with myself to this day knowing I asked her if she had any weapons in the house then doubting that I actually did and just thought that I did.

She had set on the edge of her bed and placed the gun under her chin. The bullet had torn through her palate, sinuses and then run havoc in her frontal lobe exiting her head and spraying the ceiling with blood, gore and pieces of her skull.

She was not dead.

We worked her to save her life and to suppress our feelings of guilt. We believed we were the last people to talk to her. Was there something we could have done? Said?

This is the type of thing that I lose sleep over. Not the blood or death. Not the senseless violence. It's the late at night fear that I wonder if I could have done more.....

SUCTION

Suction defined: the production of a partial vacuum by the removal of air in order to force fluid into a vacant space or to procure adhesion.

Having an item stuck in or to your body can be traumatic, but depending on how odd the item is, or its placement, the medics, nurses, and doctors may find you as hilarious and worthy of whispering about.....for years.

Our patient told us he had fallen down in the shower. What he was doing with an 8oz glass Coke bottle in the shower he couldn't really explain. His bad luck continued as he explained that when he fell on the bottle, the whole thing went neck first up his rectum. It looked like he just, had a glass inspection window installed in his asshole.

We transported him in the kneeling position, butt up in the air. Face on the stretcher, All the way to the hospital. He bemoaned his luck and misfortune and kept saying how he tried to pull it out but it was stuck. "It has suction and feels like it's pulling my guts out when I tug on it!"

We roll our patient in and present him to the doctor who does an amazing job of keeping a straight face as he hears our report. They place our patient in a cube and close the curtains. We step out to deal with paperwork and stomach pains from holding in all the laughter.

As we are composing ourselves and preparing to leave, a nurse heads into the cubicle with an ancient looking dental drill, foot petal and all. We look at each other like, "Did we really just see that?"

Then we hear the sound that has been sending chills up the spines of children and adults alike since the 1870s, the whrrrrrrr of the dental drill. Then the sound of the drill making the scratching sound as it impacts a hard object. In this case the glass bottle.

This sound is accompanied by our former patient's very high pitched voice shrieking over the sound of the drill "It's hot, it's hot!!!"

3, 2, 1 GO!!!!

As I've said many times, a bored medic is a dangerous thing. They can find mischief in the most benign places and things. Things like picking up sprint units from the mechanic shop.

It was a slow night and the shift Supervisor called my unit and asked if my partner and I could pick him up and take him to Motor Maintenance. We got him and headed over there to find that there were two brand new Taurus SHO's, freshly stickered and prepared, for the Department Director and the Operations Manager.

The Supervisor looked at me and just smiled an evil smile. "Should we?" he said. "Oh we should!" I replied.

We pulled these front wheel drive beasts out of the yard and onto the street. We set side by side with my partner in the ambulance behind us. The Supervisor rolled down his window and raised his radio up to his lips.

"Dispatch, can I get a radio check? Can you give me a count down from 5........."

Dispatch responded. "Radio check 5.....4....3....2.......1"

We hit the gas pedal like the hounds of hell were on our heels.

I've never been called a cautious driver and I do have a bit of a competitive streak in me. This caused an all-out war to win this race. We ran side by side toward the interstate on-ramp jockeying back and forth running the engines as hard as we could. By the slimmest of margins I beat him to the ramp leaving him on my rear bumper pressing for advantage.

We made it onto the three lane wide interstate and did our best to imitate a scene straight out of the Dukes of Hazard. The only thing we were missing was a barking basset hound. Our down ramp was only two exits away but we still were able to roll the speeds up into the triple digits.

I was again able to squeeze him out at the one lane down ramp holding to my fragile lead. The bottom of the ramp was a hard left turn and we took it at speed. I don't think I had ever heard of drifting back then so this panicked power slide was my introduction. I knew we had 2 blocks straight then a 90 degree right at the next red light. Once we made it there it was about a one mile straight away.

I got to the right turn in the lead but had to slow to navigate the corner in a skipping sliding manor. That bit of caution was to be my undoing.

Throwing caution, and good sense, to the wind my opponent cut the corner using the gas station as a short cut and launching himself airborne past the gas pumps and into the lead. I could just imagine the stunned look on the clerks face as a car flew past his window.

The cars being equally matched in engine displacement (if not the sanity of the drivers) held position during the last straight away. I could not squeeze anything more out of the engine to get passed him. We slid around the final turn sliding to a stop at our station and I was never able to retake the lead.

As we stepped out and away from the vehicles listening to them hiss and tick as they cooled and smelling the scent of burning brake pads I was pretty sure that we were going to need to return to motor maintenance for a rematch, I mean a repair.

~~PRISON HOOCH~~ ᗡᗡᗡᗡᗡᗡᗡᗡᗡᗡᗡᗡᗡᗡᗡᗡᗡᗡᗡᗡᗡᗡᗡᗡᗡᗡ

On my days off from the New Orleans Health Department, like many other poor medics, I worked other jobs. One of my other jobs was also as a paramedic, but for a private service. They had contracts with hospitals, nursing facilities, doctor's offices and in this case the local prison for the city of New Orleans.

Calls at the prison required more steps to get to your patient but really weren't all that different than the kind you got from the City at large. On this particular day we got a call for a possible seizure in one tier of the prison. As we are in route we get a call from dispatch advising us that they were sending another unit because they now have a report of another seizure. Hmmmmmmm......this is getting interesting.

We arrive at the prison and before we can get inside through security, dispatch is calling us again. They advise that the whole damn tier is seizing....Oh shit!

All available units are dispatched. Sure enough roughly 30 people in the tier including the 2 guards on duty are flopping like beached trout. We start an assembly line. Two men in SCBA units go in and retrieve patients we get them on a stretcher, and pass them down the line each stop on the line has a different job. Get them on oxygen, start and IV, push drugs if needed. A last stop on the line puts 2 patients in an ambulance and pair a guard with them and off they head to the hospital.

Once all the patients have been handled and we get a look around in the tier we find our seizure inducing culprit. It's not terrorists or an elaborate escape plan, its man's second oldest vice........liquor. One of the inmates had an idea for a still. He concocted a method to cook his daily helping of creamed corn and other items in an attempt to make prison hooch. He had one major flaw.

    A still is an enclosed system. It does not vent into the air. It uses pressure and collection of the fluids as they change states to make their product. Our inmate missed this step and was venting an unknown poison of creamed corn gas into the tier. This gas eventually displaced enough good air to affect everyone in the tier. I have a feeling he was not going to get a warm reception when they all returned to the cell block.

WEDGIE

Like most men I consider myself a pretty good driver, but if I am to be honest my track record probably doesn't back that statement up. I have had several mishaps in the ambulance and thought I'd share the highlights.

Tale #1

Everyone that drives knows how it is to get used to a certain vehicle. You get into something different and reach for a nonexistent shifter, or reach for a switch that is not there. I had a similar feeling as I get into a leased ambulance. My regular unit was in for warranty repairs and the company had provided us a temporary replacement. The unit was a much bigger and decked out model. I was actually really enjoying it.

We picked up a patient that wanted to go to Mercy hospital. Mercy was a smaller, older hospital with an ER on the second floor. The ramp went up to an area for unloading patients. It was basically a wedge of the hospital opened to drive through between the floors. I'd driven it 50 or 60 times. No problem.

I guess I kind of forgot that the truck I was in was bigger. I pulled up the ramp and as I entered under the roofed area you could hear the screech of the roof metal dragging against the concrete......crap.

I had to let the air out of all 6 tires and limp the truck like some wounded beast out from under to free it.

Tale #2

When I worked for New Orleans there wasn't enough Paramedics to have two in every truck. So paramedics were to handle all the patient care and not allowed to drive except to allow your partner to eat.

I regularly would tell my partners to let me drive. Let's face it the rush of driving lights and sirens is something I couldn't just leave to someone else.

We get a call while I am in the driver's seat. I flip the lights on and my young partner lectures me that he should be driving. I begin to regale him with my driving prowess and insult his youth and inexperience. I believe it went something like I've been driving in this City since you were popping zits in Junior High or something to that affect.

About the time I finished my diatribe I found a particularly narrow spot between two parked cars and wedged the unit in perfectly and when I say perfectly I mean I equally damaged my unit and both parked cars.

The only thing that decreased my embarrassment was when my young apprentice turned to me and said "Should we make a run for it?" All I did was point to the roof and the running light bar and his shoulders slumped. It was unlikely we had gone un-noticed.

PILE UP

When you think back on calls its often times difficult to remember how they originated or who you were with. It's strange the things that stick with you and why. I can remember being with Jenn and that it was an extremely foggy day. Those things don't really help limit down the days all that much but the fact that we were headed to back up another unit on a multi car pile-up on the I-10 twin spans was.

The Interstate-10 twin spans are a 5-mile section of bridges that connect the south shore (New Orleans) to the North shore (Slidell) of Lake Pontchartrain on its Eastward trek to Mississippi and states beyond. It is heavily traveled every day.

We were the second unit in route to the call. A good friend, Ruel, was in that first unit. As he was getting close he was relaying what was happening.

"We are on the bridge. Visibility is close to zero. Traffic is at a dead stop and there are already fender benders. I don't think we can get any further in the unit. We are going forward on foot." Ruel advised.

I called him directly to see where he thought our unit should head to coordinate care. He said he was about 10 cars in and hadn't found any obvious patients. The fog was extremely thick and he felt the accident could be miles long. We discussed options and decided I would use the old bridge on the state highway to cross the lake and try and approach the accident from the other direction.

I explain this plan to my partner Jenn. She is less then pleased. She is not a fan of my driving on a normal day. Today I'm telling her I am going to cross a two lane bridge in heavy fog at high speeds.

She immediately lights a cigarette.

For the next 10 minutes she will juggle between lighting one cig off the butt of the previous and saying "Oh Gawd, Oh Gawd, Oh Gawd!!" as we weave through traffic moving in both directions. She will keep one foot on the dash and one hand on the oh-shit bar doing a juggling act of swearing and smoking.

Just about the time I think Jenn will have a stroke, we reach the other side of the lake. Ruel says he is now 30 plus cars in and has found some minor injuries which he was herding back toward his unit. We start heading westbound in the eastbound lane at a crawl. The strobe lights played off the fog like a disorienting message from beyond. The only thing we can clearly see is the next stripe on the road in front of us as we inch forward like a giant colorful Pac-man.

We finally come upon the first cars in this gigantic pile-up, the catalyst that started this whole event. It's a single car accident that has rolled over. There is only one occupant and she is obviously deceased. In the heavy fog the cars just kept coming plowing one after another into each other, unable to ebb their forward momentum.

In the end there were 72 vehicles involved. 1 fatality but many more injuries both physical and emotional. Situations like this are not something that you are taught to handle. There are no steps or algorithm that walks you through it. This shows the amazing abilities of the people in the field to take the calls as they come and to be flexible and adaptive in the face of oddities, outrage, and mayhem.

Years of training and countless repetition build in you a knowledge base that allows you to read the signs and symptoms of a patient and come to a quick conclusion of what you believe is wrong so you can begin treatment. I've used this on countless patients including family and friends, but I never thought I would use it on myself.

I had been sick with the flu for more than a week and was finally feeling well enough to get back in the gym. I was dedicated to my daily Crossfit workouts and was feeling pretty guilty for missing a week. I was in the 6am class and was pushing it doing box jumps. It was hard to breath but I was not surprised….it always hurts to breath when I'm working out. It increases to a pretty intense squeeze in my chest.

I stop for a minute to catch my breath. My coach jumps my ass for slacking and I get back at it. When I finish up I am dizzy and seriously short of breath. I few minutes rest and the pain finally goes away. Being a medic and a man I do exactly what you would expect. I ignore what happened and go about my day telling no one. I'm telling myself it's just related to the flu.

I finish the day at work without further problems and settle down for the evening. Now my Wife would have me tell you fine people that I went out for a run, but if you promise not to tell her, we were having sex when I began to feel short of breath (again). My thought was "Damn that's not good".

Then the chest pain started and as classic as every book I've read, it was substernal; it was squeezing in nature and radiated to my left shoulder. I started to feel weak and light headed.

I got up quickly and rushed to the bathroom…..yep I was getting nauseous. Holy shit what is happening to me (This would be denial) I'm in the best shape of my life. This can't be happening to me…can it?

By this time my Wife is worried as you can imagine. She asks the question that wives have asked for thousands of years. "Are you alright?" and being a man I say….."I'm fine, just give me a minute."

The next thing I feel is something that is in the books and I have had patients tell it to me, but it wasn't until that very moment that I understood it. I was overwhelmed with a feeling of impending doom. I thought I was going to die!

I would later learn that I had a 95% block of the LAD (Left Anterior Descending Artery) better known in medical circles as the widow maker and that being in great physical shape may have been the only reason I didn't die.

As I stood over the sink though, I was contemplating not going to the hospital. I kept telling my wife I was fine and to just give me a minute.

In the 20 plus years we have been together we have fought and argued about a lot of things but she did something then that left no room for dispute. She left the bathroom and when she returned she had the cell phone in one hand and car keys in the other.

She said I could go in the car or she could call the ambulance that was the only choices I had. I was going no matter what. I know I'm just a dumb guy, but that sealed the deal. She drove me to the hospital.

I guess the punch line is that as we are making the final turn to the hospital I told her about the chest pain at the gym that morning and she hit the brakes so hard I thought I was going to be ejected. She cut me the stink eye and said "I just can't believe you. Are you stupid or something?" I'm going to go with or something.....it sounds better.

FLOATER

Death is not funny, but the black humor most emergency responders enjoy is a natural and vital part of their defense mechanisms. We tend to block out the horrors and find the most twisted things as funny. So when I tell you that there can be anything at all funny about a floating dead body, I ask you to trust me and maybe you will find the humor as well.

The call out for the floater was not odd. Working on the southern end of the Mississippi river brought a lot of things down to us. This was a person that had been dead for several days and had floated and bloated their way into a dock area on the river. We were sent out in a boat to retrieve the body and one of the deputies we knew, let's call him Chuck, wanted to go with us. Who are we to turn him down?

We get to the body which is pinned up against the dock. Chuck wants to be the one to use the hook to wrangle the body to the boat. You have to understand that there is a certain science to getting the body in. This flesh has soaked in water for days the internal decomposition is breaking it down from the inside also. The trick is to us the giant hook and actually snag the body between the ribs and use the strength of the skeletal system to hold him together.

Chuck did not remember any of these things.

He reached out with the hook snagging the body under an arm. He then tried to use his weight to leverage the body out of the water. This did not work. The muscles and tendons of the shoulder were so weak and water logged that they just separated and his arm popped off. To make matters worse the arm now sunk and the body being dislodged started floating away.

All we could do was make fun of Chuck for his vaudevillian destruction of the body. He was never allowed to assist us again.

WILD KINGDOM

The call is a bloody nose. We are in one of the City's housing projects. It's about 10pm and we are on the front steps of one of the residences working on our very large lady with sudden onset of walking into the wall and making her nose bleed. A true medical emergency (sarcasm). We are watching about a dozen kids running in the courtyard playing as we handle the paperwork and encourage this lady to just go inside and not to the hospital.

The change was more like a feeling. One minute everything seemed fine and then I felt like something was wrong. I look back toward the courtyard and don't see anything.....ding ding...that's it. The kids are all gone. Do you remember watching Mutual of Omaha's Wild Kingdom and all the animals would be at the watering hole? Then the predators would approach and all the other animals would vanish. That's what I felt had happened here. The kid's senses were much keener than ours and had detected the approaching danger and beat feet.

It seemed that gang members from two different groups were facing off across the courtyard we were in. Bullets started flying. I have never been called a small man so I ran back up the stoop into the solid concrete stairwell of the building. My partner was a smaller than I, so he was able to duck under the front stairs.......Our patient was obviously not on the same wave length as she laid down on the steps and started screaming, save me, save me.

Now I'm a compassionate man, sorta, sometimes. I wouldn't want to see anyone hurt at least but I was not coming out of my hiding spot to drag this large women with a nose bleed to safety.

She yells. "SAVE ME!"

I yell. "Crawl this way!"

She yells. "SAVE ME!"

I yell. "Crawl this way!"

She finally says. "I can't!"

I respond. "Then you're going to die!"

Suddenly she was struck. Not with a bullet but the ability to move and she scurried, fast as you please, up the steps in to the stairwell.

As fast as it all started it was over. My partner extricated himself from under the steps. I stood up straightened my clothes and made sure I hadn't wet myself.

Our patient then asked if we were going to take her to the hospital. We advised her that she appeared to be medically fit after seeing her sprinting abilities and we were pretty sure there was someone nearby that needed us more than her.

WATER COOLER CRUELTY

Pranks are part of the gig but sometimes they go well beyond what is considered just fun and games.

Everyone that works in public service at some time or another hates the person on the other end of the radio that tells you where to go and what to do. Your dispatcher can be your best friend or the bane of your existence.

A paramedic to remain nameless was very unhappy with the dispatchers. He felt he was wronged by them on a regular basis and his loathing grew and grew.

He finally decided to act on this hate.

One of the many drugs that are carried on the ambulance is Lasix. This drug is designed to remove fluid from the body. In the simplest explanation possible it makes you pee.

Our culprit decided that the way to get back at his nemesis dispatchers was to place this drug in the dispatcher's water cooler. Did I say that he put A LOT of Lasix in this water cooler?

The three people working in the dispatch room would drink a glass of cool refreshing water. The water would enter their system and the urge to pee would stir in them. They would relieve themselves. Then they would return back to work. This would lead at some point to them suddenly having a feeling of thirst that they couldn't seem to quench. So what did they do? Yep, they drink more water!

The end result was at least one trip to the emergency room, several dehydrated dispatchers and one medic looking for gainful employment.

LIKE MOTHS TO A FLAME

The events, actions and emotional time known as hurricane Katrina have filled many books. I could probably write one myself, but this isn't the place. The story I want to tell here is more about a very specific moment in time.

I was working as a cop and a medic when hurricane Katrina struck. I stayed in the city to do what I felt needed doing, but as a person that likes order, even craves it in things, I along with most everyday people were not prepared for the world after the storm passed.

The people in public service were still in uniform, following rules, hell I had on a starched shirt on day one. The thugs and miscreants had no problem realizing that the world had temporarily stopped rotating. That the rules no longer applied.

It was just a few nights after the storm. My team was working security for the fire department and EMS units. Everyone had been stationed on the Westbank of the Mississippi and as calls came out across the 350 square miles of city, the fire and EMS units would head out taking a 4-man security force (we had, had people trying to steal or vandalize units and harass responders). A fire unit went out on a call in the middle of the night. I had been sleeping but heard them go out. Shortly after they arrived on the scene one of the guys called back to the CP (Command Post) asking for some back up. They said it was a big fire and they were concerned about crowd control.

I jumped in my gear and was out the door with my partner in minutes. We were running around in a world with hardly no activity on the streets, no power, and no lights. The amount of activity moving around was so low as to be non-existent. The feeling of aloneness was overpowering.

We topped the Crescent City Connection Bridge over the Mississippi river and off in the distance was one light, fire light, at the location we were headed to. It was the only point bright enough to identify. An eerie orange and yellow beacon in the darkness of a city that we were unsure was going to survive the next few days.

We slowed as we looked and the only thought that clearly resonated with me was that the fire was like a message, it would be the only thing visible for miles, and much like a moth to the flame, and this fire would draw all the people that were happy with the fall of the City. The wolves, the hyenas the mentally imbalanced would all be drawn to it looking to be dazzled by the lights and feed on its energy.

It was in that moment that I understood. I knew then that this was more than a fight for a few miles of flooded real estate. It was a battle for the soul of a people. A guerrilla war to save the cultural heart of the City I loved. In the end we lost a few of the battles but I think we won the war.

POINTE NOIRE

     I took a job that most would find very strange. I signed on to be a medic on an oil platform in Africa. What can I say, the money was right and I have enjoyed traveling before. The plan was to have me travel with the rest of the Americans that would make crew change for the 28 day on and 28 day off shift rotation. Some hiccup in the visa process and communication between my company and the main group caused me to be two days behind and traveling alone.

     First leg of the flight is New Orleans to New York. A pretty normal trip. I'm in my regular travel outfit, jeans, a polo shirt, and an old sports coat. I find this to be the perfect travel clothes because it's pretty comfortable and the jacket has lots of pockets for all the travel items I have. It can also be used as a cover on the plane if it's cold. I think it is casual but professional enough to get by in any situation.

     I land at LaGuardia and realize that I need to get from domestic flights to international. I first have to collect all my baggage including checked bags. I am sure there is some sort of skyway or underground people mover to do this. I never found it. I ended up outside walking down the road dragging my bags. I'd like to blame this on their signage or airport officials giving me bad directions…….but I can't, it was all me. I was just lost.

     I finally reach the International Terminal, now sweaty and huffing out of breath. I get my requisite grope from TSA as I make my third pass through security so far. I recheck my bags find my concourse and am just in time to board my flight to Paris.

     Now it's worth mentioning at this point that I left New Orleans at about 1pm. My flight from New

York left around 5pm. This would mean my flight to Paris would be an overnighter, arriving in Paris at 6am. The plan was to sleep as much as possible. So much for the plan. I was keyed up and didn't get nearly enough sleep.

Arrival in Paris is uneventful. I spend a few minutes diagnosing the signage to figure out where I need to go to find my flight to Africa. I work my way across the airport to the main hub of the international concourse and low and behold I find a bastion to capitalism. Starbucks! Now I am not normally a fan of the Chief mate of the HMS Pequod, but I am a junkie for coffee. It's 6 in the morning and I am going to be in Africa for a month. I'll take an extra-large with an extra shot, thank you.

I lug my bags and my coffee to my gate. I check in and get a seat to wait and people watch. The other passengers are an odd mix. I see a few others like me, European or American guys, dressed casual in what I can assume is the oil field look. I also see what I assume is African business men. Suits, ties, well-groomed but from a westerner's eye, out of date. It was kind of like looking at Christmas pictures of family from 20 years ago. The last group were obviously people local to where we were headed. They dressed in what appeared to be traditional clothing' Ladies in colorful one piece dresses and men in light fabric tops and color pants. It reminded me very much of what I saw in the Caribbean, another hot humid place.

We board the flight and take off to make the eight and a half hour flight that will remove me from what I think of as the modern world. We are headed to Pointe Noire, Congo.

As we make our final approach I can see the city below. Two things strike me. First it's a very large city. It seems to spread out over dozens of miles. Second, it's appears low to the ground, like it is trying not to intrude on the sky. I see hardly any buildings over two stories tall. I can see the coast line of a beautiful beach buffeted by the Atlantic and off in the distance, mountains, deep inland in the jungle.

As we get lower and line up for landing the next thing that strikes me is the obvious poverty. I have traveled a lot and seen a fair piece of the world so it's not a new thing to see but it's on such a large scale here. The plywood huts and garbage piles. The dirt paths and general rundown look of things.

The landing is uneventful but the views out the window continue to elicit trepidation. As we pass what passes for a terminal I see four Mig 21 jet fighters emblazoned with the Congolese flag. I'm not sure what those are protecting this country from but in counter pose to the poverty, a picture is starting to form about what kind of place I've landed.

We role toward the terminal but stop short. They push a set of rolling stairs out to our 767 jet and we are ushered out onto the hot evening tarmac. They herd us across the airfield to the only structure close, a two story building that I assume is the terminal. The first floor customs area is where we are brought and the process of entering the country begins.

I of course enter the line for visitors which seems to be the majority of the people. The local's line is very short in comparison. As we work our way to the desk I see that there is the traditional stop to stamp your passport and check your visa but there is an another stop after that.

I clear the passport check and the second stop is health records inspection and in broken English I am informed that mine are not up to standards. Now, I work for an international company of doctors. They stuck me a dozen times before I traveled. I know this is bullshit. Sure enough as I watch others going through this check I see they look at your shot records and then rub their index finger and thumb together in the obviously international symbol for money. I have a five dollar bill in my pocket and nothing else! I hope he is cheap. I place the five in my shot records and hand it to him. Like a magician the Franklin vanishes and I am waved through.

    The next room I enter is a madhouse. It's the baggage claim. The room is basically a barn, its upper eaves are open for air circulation. The door at the runway end has a mechanical luggage conveyor sticking through it and our baggage is being pumped in to the room making its way around on the belt in its never ending circle. People are hollering in several languages (none of them English) others holding signs with people's names or company names on it trying to summon them.

    I elbow my way up to the conveyor belt to hunt up my luggage. I'm also pretty sure I'm seeing things. I see luggage, a few boxes, but also a bunch of odd shit like gallon bottles of liquid (assorted colors), sacks of rice, and a tricycle. It was the weirdest collection of things I'd ever seen coming off a plane.

    My rather pedestrian black suitcase finally came around and now I had to get my luggage cleared through customs. First problem is lack of communication. They spoke French and I didn't. Second problem was that I was out of cash. I got the full baggage inspection due to my lack of funds. Bribes are only taken in cash it seems.

    I am finally released and head to the entrance/exit door. There are no soda stands or snack kiosks it's just very utilitarian. Outside I find dozens of people standing right around the doors all yelling and trying to interest me in different items.

There are things such as taxi people and also some folks trying to hawk phone cards. There were also people selling food and a few selling private time with their women. This was all at the front doors of the airport!

It takes me over an hour to hunt down someone that can speak enough English to find my driver. My driver grabs my luggage and pushes his way through the throng of people all while hollering at them. He loads me into his van and off we go through the city streets.

The city is mostly cinder block construction with lots of very small businesses along the main potholed thoroughfare. The stores we see through the windows have only a few dozen items on the shelves showing how difficult it is to get supplies. We pass a bar that has a large crowd spilling out into the street. They have a projector putting the soccer game up on the outside wall and all the crowd is into it.

There are very few streetlights and then only at the round-abouts. Spaced in the middle of all this poor hoard are these tall walled compounds that are obviously designed to keep the unwashed masses out. You can see manicured lawns past heavy iron gates as we drive by.

My destination is the Hotel Palm Beach along the white sands of the Atlantic. It is also a walled compound and caters exclusively to Westerners. The large cabana restaurant has several people eating. They appear to be European and Middle Eastern. The hotel has a large beautiful pool with a slide. It seems so out of place after the city I've just emerged from.

I am checked in by someone with a better grasp of English than my grasp of French which isn't saying much. The entire transaction is mostly done via sign language. My room is nice. It is a very good attempt to mimic an American hotel room. It is kind of the equivalent of Chinese food in America. It's close but obviously not the same as the real thing and it is probably one of the nicest places in the entire country. I turn on the TV and the only channel not in French is Aljazeera.....sigh. I am lucky enough to video chat with the wife and then I'm off to bed. I wish I could talk to my son but in New Orleans he is still in school while I'm headed to bed in Africa.

I wake up in this strange, vaguely unsettling hotel room (it just doesn't feel right to my American senses) and head to breakfast. It is also oddly disturbing in its normality. It is a classic European breakfast. Cured meats, French breads, soft scrambled eggs and tea....... damn tea. I sooo wanted coffee.

I check out using the reverse of the sign language from last night and get in my ride to get me to the heliport. The city is less scary but equally as depressing as the bright light shines into the cracks and the third world nature is bracingly obvious.

Armed militia are on street corners. Peddlers pushing carts with various foods for sale. It's humbling when you see what other parts of the world are like and how good you have it back home. It makes the phrase 1st world problems seem so ironic once you have a true context to put it against.

I reach the heliport and 'surprise!' It the same airport I left last night. I guess I should have seen that coming. I get signed in and go through the bi-lingual safety orientation and then get ushered out to the flight line.

I am momentarily staggered when I see my ride. It's a Bell 205 but that's not the term I think of when I see it. It's a Huey to me. A UH-1D to be exact. The helicopter that made its debut in the mid-60s and I had the honor of being a crew chief on in the 80s.

What staggers me is this is 2014, in Africa, meaning this bird has been in operation for about 50 years! I load up taking a seat I am extremely familiar with and look forward over the shoulder of the pilot. I see our GPS unit. It is the latest model......from the sporting goods store! It is a handheld hiker's model and it is Velcro attached to the dashboard of the helicopter.

My thoughts are that after traveling 7000 miles I'm going to be lost at sea when we have to ditch from a 50 year old helicopter.

KATRINA TEARS

It had been nearly two weeks since Katrina hit the city and compounded with the man-made failures of the levees some areas were still holding water.

I had seen many sad, gruesome or otherwise depressing things in these days, but I had a job to do and there was no time to sit back and work through my emotions. My family was safe and all out of the city. I had visited my Parent's and Sister's house in Chalmette a week earlier but the water had been so high that they were not accessible. I had cruised by in a boat and saw that the water was still up to the top of the door sills.

I was going back today to survey my family's homes and report to them. I visited my parent's one story home first and the destruction was total. The house recently had over 9 foot of water in it. It had receded now, but the inside of the house looked like it was the drum of a demonic washing machine, tossing things around in tumble cycle. It, like all the others around it, was a total loss.

I moved on to my sister's house. She lived in a very nice two story home with her husband and my two nieces. The water had been violent enough to pull the doors off their hinges and throw everything on the first floor topsy turvy. The water line in their house was 14 foot off the ground.

I made my way upstairs to find that the water had been high enough to wash over most everything close to the ground on that level. The mattresses and long hanging clothes were all ruined.

I walked in to my nieces' room to see slime on the carpet, mold growing on stuffed animals and toys.

I had witnessed death, depravity and a general decline in humanity over the weeks but had stayed strong and positive. The sight of their toys ruined and forever taken from them was my emotional tipping point. A lumped formed in my throat as I rushed out the house but I couldn't stop the tears from coming.

I cried for the things they had lost. I cried for the change that was thrust on them and all of us. I cried for that piece of innocence that they would lose because of this tragedy. I cried for my unborn son and the different world he would call normal. I cried for myself because all I wanted to do was protect my family and I was unsure if I would be able to in this new reality.

LAWYERS

When working as a city Rescue tech your normal calls are from auto accidents, the occasional house with bars needs cutting, but there are always those calls that seem to have a desire to be different.

The call comes in as a man with his hand trapped in a Coke machine. It's on the 23rd floor of One Shell Square, the tallest building in New Orleans and one of the places with the highest rental prices for offices. I'm directed to the loading bay were I lug a set of jaws and the power pack for it as well as a few other tools and board the service elevator. I'm guessing some poor bastard was working on a machine and got a finger stuck in the mechanism.

What I find when I reach the floor is not what I expected. There is a circle of old white men around the Coke machine. All with gray hair and in very expensive looking suits from the looks of them. I part the sea of suits to find a young black guy also in a very nice suit on his knees in front of the machine. His right hand is buried almost to the elbow in the drink shoot. I ask what happened and he says that he put his money in and he heard the soda come down but it never came out, so he reached up to grab it and once he got his hand around the can he couldn't get his arm out.

"Did anyone here attempt to help?" I asked. He said no they were all just standing around gawking saying how he should sue. He didn't argue because he was the newest and the only black attorney at the firm.

By this time the collected group was getting a little grumpy peppering me with questions about when I was going to cut up the machine and free the young lawyer.

I stood up and asked for everyone's attention. Once they were all focused on me I stepped to the side of the machine and unplugged it. The lawyers hand immediately came out along with his Coke. I then asked the collected crowd who at the firm the City should send my rescue bill to, for services rendered. The room emptied pretty quickly.

NOTE TO THE CORONER

At one point in time we not only responded to the calls for medical service but if it was determined that they were deaths that required autopsies we were tasked with transporting the bodies to the morgue. This normally didn't cause us any problem other than maybe the smell but on occasion accidents happen that need clarification.

We were working an auto accident with two fatalities. Both of our patients would be transported to the morgue. We placed the first one on a wooden spine-board (now you know how long ago this was) and placed him on the bench seat. It wasn't like he was going to need medical care where he was going. We took the stretcher to the second and lifted him up placing him on the stretcher. When we lifted the stretcher up to full height we realized we had him on the stretcher backwards (head to the rear). Again, no bigee, he wouldn't mind.

We roll him to the back of the truck and begin the procedure of loading the stretcher into the back. My poor dead patient's arms fall off the stretcher swinging out from his sides just as I'm shoving him in the back. He can't seem to catch a break....well maybe.

I catch his left arm against the door of the truck and hear a loud POP and CRACK all we needed was snap and we would have the set.

Sure enough on examining him he now has a broken arm to add to the things that killed him in the car accident. Shit what do we do? Suddenly my partner no longer felt that this was a "we" situation. I was on my own.

My first thought was to pretend it didn't happen, hoping the Coroner would write it off as more trauma from the accident. The problem with that is if he didn't buy it as an injury from the accident, and he went all CSI, it would appear that foul play had happened.

    I know!! I'll write a note.

Dear Dr. Minyard,

In loading the deceased into the unit for transport a technical malfunction caused his left humorous to be fractured during loading. I regret any complications I have caused in regards to this case.

                         Sincerely,

                         B.J.

    I pinned the note the shirt of the deceased and delivered him to the morgue making no mention to the night attendant about the note.

    About a week later I received an envelope from the coroner's office. When I opened it my letter was inside with the added message written below.

You broke his arm on the ambulance door. Not the first time I've seen that. Thanks for being honest.

                             Frank M.

HURRICANE ANDREW

The plan was to stay and ride out the storm. We weren't going to respond on anything. It would be too dangerous. That was the plan. What ended up happening was of course totally different.

As hurricane Andrew came on shore late that night my partner and I were safe and dry in my apartment in Violet. It was decided that we would hold the lower half of St. Bernard from my house since it was an all cinder block building.

Dispatch asked that I call them on the phone. They had a problem. They said that the Yscloskey bridge (look it up on Google) operator had seen a shrimp boat break free of its moorings and it was heading at the bridge. The operator panicked and attempted to raise the bridge over the boat to let it pass underneath. Her timing was poor and the wing nets on the boat got tangled in the bridge railing. Now the bridge couldn't go up or down and since this was the only way on or off of the lower portion of the Parish something needed to be done.

From warm and dry to cold and wet in a flash. We drove toward the bridge being beaten by the rain and buffeted by the winds. Our swirling emergency lights looked eerie against the sheets of rain.

On our arrival the problem was obvious the wire cables on the nets were hooked on the rails of the bridge. Only problem the bridge was 20 feet up in the air in the middle of a hurricane.

My partner and I decided that one of us would need to climb up there and cut the cables while the other directed the bridge operator in what to do. It was decided in the most democratic way possible who would go.

Rock, Paper, Scissors.

I still think he cheated!

I grabbed the bolt cutters from the trunk and went to the bridge structure. Crap this is going to suck.

It did.

I held tight and worked my way up the iron frame trying to stay as close as I can to the bridge as the wind tries to rip me free. I make it up to the bridge deck and have to walk hunched over to make headway in the torrent of weather. I find the cable and start cutting it free. When I get to the last strands, I radio my partner to have the bridge raised. Pop, the last line goes and the bridge jumps up fast knocking me to my knees. The boat, now free, goes under the bridge and drifts down the bayou to run aground. I take the ride all the way to the top holding tightly to the railing. It is scary and exhilarating all at the same time. The power of the storm is all encompassing.

The ride ends as I am brought back down and I realize I am soaked to the bone. Time to go back and hope we ride out the rest of this storm in peace.

GRAND PRIX DU MARDI GRAS

A spectacle to be seen, formula one racing in the streets of New Orleans. It is also a nightmare for city services. The race rendered the city divided and made travel difficult. Ambulances were based in zones to attempt to make the best overall coverage possible.

The problem with this is that life goes on in the Big Easy for better or worse and resources are always stretched thin so an event like this means we have to find unique solutions to problems.

I had heard a call come out for a school bus accident. The unit got on the scene reported that it was simply a bump and that they would handle it....phew...that could have been a nightmare. The unit is on the scene for about 30 minutes and I hear them clear the scene with 22 patient refusals of care. Although that seemed odd I didn't think much of it at that moment.

Time past, as it's known to do, and dispatch contacted my partner and I. We were informed that NOPD had arrived at the bus accident, finally, and was concerned about all these kids. They wanted us to go over and check things out since we were now the closest unit.

As we pull up, I see a school bus full of kids jumping and scurrying around. The bus driver was standing outside the bus talking to the Police Officer. I walk up and talk with them and find that the previous unit had gotten the bus driver to sign a report refusing medical care on behalf of all of the kids. Unfortunately that's not how it works and the cop knew it. I knew it and the bus driver was quickly realizing that he didn't want it to be his responsibility. Crap.

I walk on the bus and started talking to the kids they are all middle school kids around 12 years old. No one is claiming injury they are all enjoying the adventure of this accident.

I call the doctor at med control and explain my problem. "I've got a bus load of minors with no parents or guardians on site. Only person I have is a bus driver. No one is claiming that they are hurt but they are minors." I inform him.

We are in quite a quandary. Doc makes the command decision that they should all be brought to the hospital to be medically cleared the problem is that they need to be immobilized as protocol demands. Dispatch was obviously listening in to my call because they cut in and tell me there are no other ambulances to assist me. Crap, Crap.

This is the part of the story where I made a command decision of my own, without the benefit of management's assistance. In hindsight I can see the problems with my plan but at the time it seemed perfectly logical.

I had my partner gather every C-collar, sheet, towel and roll of tape he could dig up. I told the kids we were going to have a little fun and games and take a ride. I then started making C-collars out of sheets and taping the kids to their seats.

It took maybe 15 minutes to duck tap the 22 kids to their seats. It was a work of art. I had the ambulance get in front of the bus and the NOPD car in the rear. I showed the bus driver my CDL and told him to get out of my seat.....I'm driving.

Our little parade starts heading with lights and sirens toward the hospital. I call the hospital back and advise that I'm on my way with a bus load of kids and to meet me on the ramp of the emergency room. I'm guessing with the race in town someone was listening in on our channels because as I made the final turn in my big yellow ambu-bus I was shocked to see two camera men filming my approach to the ramp. Standing on the ramp were the Doctors and Nurses I requested as well as my Supervisor and the Director of Operations. She was accompanied by a City Councilman. Crap, crap and crap.

I pull the bus onto the ER ramp, push in the air brakes Shshhhsssssss and swing the handle to open the bus doors. The docs and nurses come on board and start talking to the kids. My supervisor comes on and looks at me with a huge shit eating grin and says "I would suggest you stay on this bus as long as possible She's (the Director) pretty pissed." Seems she was not a fan of my ingenuity in patient transport.

She got the final laugh. She couldn't dress me down in front of the camera so her solution was more elegant. She made me write 22 individual patient transport reports and one refusal for the driver. All while still running regular calls. I ended up a couple of hours late with everyone that past me shaking their heads and laughing. So much for ingenuity.

RESCUING RAYMOND

There are those people in your life that always leave a mark. They are the ones that would be there for you in any situation and you would gladly stand at their side when the going got tough. Raymond was one of those kind of friends. Over the years our lives had taken different paths and I hadn't been in contact with him in sometime. He was still working as a paramedic for the City and I was working as a tactical team leader for the state.

In the aftermath of Hurricane Katrina, I had found my old world and my new world thrust back together. I was in charge of two tactical teams that were tasked with providing security to the Fire and Health Department both. They were stationed at the same compound we were and we would go as security on scenes when they would venture out.

I had heard stories from the other medics that Raymond and his dog Nikko had been with them at the Health Department Offices when the water started rising and that he and Nikko had swam to Delgado about 2 miles away to reach higher ground but when rescue came they didn't want to take his dog so he refused to go stating he would swim back to the office. That was the last the others had seen of him.

In a rare minute of downtime I was approached by one of the medics who was very excited and animated. He said that one of the Fire Dept. rescue teams had been in the area of Esplanade (which is near the Health Dept. station house) and described someone that looked like Raymond and he had a big dog with him. He figured it had to be him and could I get a team together to go find him. My answer was immediate, "Let's roll."

I got another one of my Tac team guys and a couple of volunteers to run the boat for us. We towed our 16 foot flat boat behind the police car and headed from the dry Westbank across the river to the flooded combat zone known as downtown New Orleans.

We traveled on to the elevated portion of I-10 and backed the boat down an interstate on-ramp using the angle to launch the boat into the flooded area below. We boarded and headed out in to the city.

We first attempted to go down a large main street called Orleans Ave. This was a relatively open street and we figured we would be able to navigate well. What we didn't count on was as we passed the Lafitte house projects someone in a third floor window started taking shots at us. It was a small caliber pistol so his aim was lousy but if it would have hit any of us we would still be dead. My partner and I shielded the 2 others in the boat and returned a little suppressive fire at the building. I'm pretty sure all we did was kill the red brick of the building but I do know the shooting at us stopped.

We felt getting off this main drag would be a good idea so we moved over one block to St. Ann. This was much slower going due to debris. There were cars sunk in the street and furniture floating down the road. One house we passed had the putrid smell of decay and I was 100% sure there was a dead body inside but that wasn't our mission today.

We made it up to Broad St. which is a natural high ridge in the city. We followed along it until we reached Esplanade Ave. The water at Broad and Esplanade was just a couple of inches deep so we had to get out the boat slide it over the high spot and relaunch as the water got deeper again on the other side.

We really didn't know what we were looking for or where to look specifically. Figuring he might see us or we would get lucky. We cruised down Esplanade watching for anything. I spotted a dog on a porch on a side street and we decided to check it out. The house was one of the typical New Orleans houses that are built up off the ground for ventilation and in this case protection from flooding. The water was about 3 feet deep but this house was dry.

I recognized Nikko right away and right behind him was Raymond. He looked a bit disheveled and fatigued but over all looked good. As I was telling him we were here to rescue him I could see the mischievous glint in his eyes just as the two twentysomething gypsy looking girls came out of the house only slightly dressed. Ray informed me that he had been staying here "helping out" and he wasn't quite ready for rescue yet. We told him where we were based and he was happy to take the extra food and water we carried.

As we prepared to leave he asked if I had any dip because he was out. For the life of me I am not sure why I gave the guy marooned with two pretty girls my last three tins of Skoal..... I guess that's what friends are for.

STRESSED

I will admit to being a task master and general difficult medic to work with. I have my methods for doing things and am not happy if things are altered or don't go my way. This can make it tough on my partners when I act like an asshole.

My partner Frank and I received a call for a cardiac arrest at a private home. It was the family member of a Police officer.

Now Frank was easily excitable at the time. He hadn't been in the business that long, so when we got on the scene to a very animated Police Officer wanting us to do anything to help his family member out, I think it frazzled his nerves. Me hollering for him to move his ass faster probably didn't help either.

It was definitely a cardiac arrest. I sent Frank for a spine board so we could quickly get our patient into the truck. He comes back with a board but no straps. Crap. I have the cop and his family telling us to hurry up, so we get the patient on the board then onto the stretcher. Frank is pushing the stretcher so fast and hard I think he is going to run me over. He is so amped up. We get to the truck and I climb in so that I can get to the head of the stretcher. Frank slides the stretcher in and is closing the rear doors before the stretcher locks into place.

I'm screaming and cursing like drill sergeant on the first day of boot camp. Frank jumps in the driver's seat and the Police hit their lights and sirens to lead the way. I heard the truck going in to drive and I'm pretty sure he smashed the gas pedal through the floor. I am sitting on the floor when this happens attempting to place a breathing tube in my patient.

The vehicle lurches forward accelerating and suddenly my patient is rolling toward the back doors. OH SHIT!! The stretcher wasn't locked in place. It struck the back doors and I flinched knowing my stretcher and my patient were going to fly out the back door and land on the hood of the now second police car we had escorting us.

Thanks to all that is holy, that it did not pop the doors open. I scream a string of profanities to Frank about the stretcher and he does what was a natural reaction. He hit the brakes. The stretcher rolls back towards me, over my leg and strikes the stops. The patient slides forward half off the stretcher landing in my lap. Crap. I scream that my patient is riding me like my girlfriend!

Now this goes on, back and forward, for miles with the patient sliding, the stretcher rolling, and me screaming and cursing. Frank just keeps telling me "I hear ya." Which I can only assume means "Fuck you, you loud mouth asshole!" in his language. Who could blame him.

As we make the turn into the hospital my last uttered demand was that he better have his ass at the back doors before the truck stops rolling.

I was kind of an asshole.......

DEATH FROM ABOVE

We have all heard the bible saying to turn the other cheek and as I have grown more mature I see the wisdom in that. When I was younger...... not so much. Getting payback was a necessary thing. That tit for tat had to be satisfied.

I was in the passenger seat dozing against the door, my partner was driving and we had a third rider. He was one of the Air Force Pararescue men (PJs) in town to train with us. The military figured back then that we had more gunshot wounds for them to practice on than anywhere else.

One of the other units was manned by Reggie (driving), Lance (passenger seat), and a female third rider (in the back of the unit). They pulled up next to our passenger side at a red light. Reggie stepped out of his door and opened my door causing me to flail my arms and legs in an effort to not fall out into the street. They then took off. I was embarrassed and a bit annoyed on being dumped from the truck.

We knew where they were headed. There was an abandoned construction site with an old crane. All the units knew it as a place you could be out of the eye of Joe public and hang out.

I tell my partner to go after them. I will say that I had no idea what was going through my mind or why I did what I did next, but as they say hindsight is 20/20. I didn't want to just lean out my door and get him so I climbed out of the passenger seat and back into the rear of the unit. Our PJ and I discussed options quickly and it was decided I should climb out of the back of the unit and get on the roof.........while moving down the street.

I opened the back doors and with his help I climbed up onto the roof. The PJ told my partner to get on the side of the other unit if he could. By this time we were coming down an off ramp and were slowing. At that very moment I saw how close we were to the unit and knew they might see me, so I did the dumbest thing ever. I jumped from the roof of my unit and landed on theirs. I landed and laid flat as we made the final turns into our secluded construction lot.

When we come to a stop Reggie opens his door and begins to step out. I could see that he was focused on the passenger seat of my truck looking for me. I do my best "Creature crouch" and reach down with one arm and grab Reggie by the face. He freaks falling back into the truck. Lance on the passenger side saw something reach down and grab his partner. He falls out the truck on the other side. It was panic and bedlam. The thing that broke through was my killing myself laughing on the roof of the unit. That's one medic monster they won't soon forget.

TROLL

Now I can't claim to have been present for this story. Every bit of the information is second hand from those I worked with, but the tale is funny enough that I felt I would be remiss if I didn't include it.

There are some patients that become regulars. Either due to their medical conditions or in many cases their ability to manipulate the system to their advantage. These are the people that know, if they have the right complaint when they dial 9-1-1 you can't refuse to send them a unit. I have seen them ride to the hospital and walk right out because it was just a covenant way to get to where they needed to go.

We have a term for these people TROLLS

Terrible

Ridiculous

Obnoxious

Low

Life

Scum

So this particular TROLL called so frequent that dispatch just gave you his name. He was regularly drunk, homeless, smelled and was a general pain in the ass (see how his nick name suited him?). He averaged 6 or 7 ambulance rides a week.

He was a nuisance and quickly becoming a danger to other people. If you were tied up on a call with him and someone else needed a unit they would have to wait no matter how serious the problem was.

Something had to give and the medics decided it would be in their best interest to give in. A collection was started. Everyone was urged to pony up a few dollars. Once the money was in, a bus ticket was purchased, and our TROLL was brought to the bus station given a couple of hospital egg salad sandwiches for the ride, and a one way ticket to Houston. He was told he had won a contest. He was kind of drunk so he didn't catch on at first. A fond farewell party was thrown .....After he left.

A blissful period of time passed where the TROLL did not call and torture the poor medics, but as with all good things they come to an end. Dispatch called a unit and informed them that the TROLL was back! How could this be?

When the crew met up with the TROLL they inquired as to why he had returned. He said that he was put on a bus and sent home. He also had a note for whoever sent him to Houston. It said, we don't want him we are sending him back. Next time it will be C.O.D. signed, Houston Medics.

CODE 3 CLUB

Yep, it's what you think it is. We all know the mile high club is sex in a plane over a mile up. This is the medic's version.

Wikipedia defines CODE 3 as Life-threat response. Emergency traffic, or simultaneous use of lights and siren required in order to achieve a rapid response. This allows the responding unit to ignore jurisdictional traffic laws, but does not allow the responding unit to operate without due regard to safety.

That pretty much sums it up what code 3 is. The Code 3 club would be sex of some sort in the back of an ambulance traveling under code 3 conditions. Do I have your attention yet?

So, as you can guess, every male medic at the very least (and quite a few female medics) were constantly trying to earn membership in this mystical club.

My first encounter with the Code 3 club was not as part of a couple trying to join. I was asked to be the driver of the unit.......Yep that's how it works......

The amorous couple got in the back and start warming up. I already know my job is to kill about 10 minutes and to monitor the radio then get in the cab and get on the highway making the lights and siren ad some ambiance and cover to the moaning noises.

The problem with being the driver for this is focus, and as Mr. Miyagi says my focus needs more focus. It's very hard to pay attention to the traffic you're weaving thru when you look in your mirror and see titties bouncing to the rhythm of the potholes I'm hitting.

As we speed down the road I continue to split my attention between the road and the mirror. This balance in my head seems an acceptable balance, in reality, not so much.

During one long glance into the mirror I struck the curb fairly hard. I am pretty sure that curb was new. I didn't remember it being there. I swerved then causing the rear wheels to smack the curb. Between the hits and the swerving I had thrown the couple off the stretcher onto the floor. She had let out a squeal that I am pretty sure had nothing to do with pleasure. He had bounced his head off the floor and was looking rather pale almost as pale as her bare breasts, I mean if I would have looked and I'm not saying I did……much.

It goes without saying that the mood had been ruined and that it was unlikely I would be asked by them (or anyone else) to assist in the future.

HEAVY BREATHING

In New Orleans the saying goes if you don't like the weather wait 10 minutes. That may be a bit of an exaggeration but the weather can change pretty fast and become fairly violent at times.

It had been an extremely heavy storm that day that had flooded parts of the city. One of these areas was an elderly assisted living building on St. Charles Ave. It's fourteen stories tall and had, had some flooding in the basement causing the elevator to short out. Our patient, as Murphy's Law would ensure, was on the fourteenth floor. Dispatch was nice enough to send a second unit to help my partner and I out. The four of us started up the stairs with the cardiac monitor, paramedic med bag, stair-chair and oxygen bottle in tow. The chief complaint of our patient was shortness of breath.

I won't bore you with the trip up but it was obvious that the four of us were not athletes, not in the least. We were better drinkers then stair climbers. Needless to say, we were winded just getting the gear up there.

Our patient was a tall man 6 foot 5 or so. Obviously in the early stages of Congestive Heart Failure. We begin our routine getting him on the monitor, giving him some oxygen and checking his vitals.

Son of a bitch!

We forgot the stethoscope and blood pressure cuff on the first floor. To hell with it! He is obviously sick I put my ear against his chest and can hear the fluid just fine as far as blood pressure......He has one.

We get him secured to the stair chair, a collapsible chair with small wheels, after starting an IV and giving him some medicine to help remove the fluid from his system. We now have to figure out how to carry him, the chair, the monitor, the oxygen and hold the IV bag all while traveling down 14 flights of stairs.

The juggling act was slow and painful as we inched our way down. Our patient was such a nice guy. He kept apologizing to us. I asked if he was the one that filled the basement with water. He said no. I replied, "Then you have nothing to be sorry for." "This is our job even if we don't look like we know what we're doing, we do,.....I swear."

Somewhere around the 5th floor the medicine we gave our patient kicked in. He peed all over the stair-chair......and my boots. He of course apologized again....

After what felt like eons we reached the first floor. We got our patient into the unit and were ready to head to the hospital. Being it was only a few blocks away I immediately got on the phone with the Emergency room.

I was still so out of breath and I could only get a couple of words at a time out as I'm trying to give a patient report. The ER nurse kept asking me to repeat. Then she started asking if I was O.K. My patient starts laughing and coughing. I'm out of breath and laughing. The patient then asks if I wanted him to finish the report.

~~THANKSGIVING~~

    Now working in public service pretty much guarantees that you'll have to work weekends and holidays and as a whole the holidays are pretty laid back days. I have always found Thanksgiving to be the slowest of all. In most cases good will wins out and it's a happy affair but there are always exceptions.

    I was working as a patrol officer for the local Sheriff's Office on Thanksgiving, and up until then it had been very peaceful as everyone settled into their tryptophan comas. The silence was broken as dispatch sent me to a home for a 103D (domestic disturbance). The call originated from a neighbor who said they could hear yelling and dishes breaking.

    I cruise on over to the residence and pull up one house before the one that the disturbance was at. I tell dispatch I have arrived and prepare to step out. This is when things got odd.

    The front door flies open and a roasted turkey, platter and all, comes sailing out the house and bounces across the front lawn. As I get out my unit and approach the door the mashed potatoes and green peas follow the turkey in this culinary skeet shoot.

    I step to the door and have to dodge a flying pie. I think for a minute I'm in a Charlie Chaplin movie. I hold out my hands in the international symbol for; "Don't hit me with flying holiday fare and step in the house." The food wielding demon is the lady of the house. Her husband is sitting in a recliner watching football and showing very little emotion about the current situation.

I ask her what's going on. She begins to tell me how she had fixed Thanksgiving dinner for the two of them and had put a considerable amount of time into it. She had laid it all out on the table and had called him to come in and eat. He refused to come to the table wanting her to bring him a plate so he could watch the game. That was the point I believe when the yelling and screaming was heard by the neighbor.

In the end the only thing that got her to calm down was when I asked her "Did you at least save a plate for yourself?" Her mouth fell open. So much for the feast and the giving of thanks.

S.I.D.S.

Sudden Infant Death Syndrome is something that, as a medic, you dread to your core. I know I will never feel the way the parents of these babies feel and I would never begin to feel that my emotions on these calls approaches theirs, but I want you to know about it from the medics perspective.

The call is always in the morning, early in the morning, that's when most deaths are noticed. Dispatch calls and says you have an unresponsive infant. They say they are not sure if the baby is breathing. You feel that sinking feeling in the pit of your stomach and you put on as much speed as you can hoping beyond hope that it's something you can combat. Thinking about your own kids and then locking those thoughts away because you know you'll need to focus and can't let your emotions get in the way.

You get to the address and many times one of the parents comes running out to you carrying the child. They are so desperate for hope of any kind, they come to you, seeing you as the answer to a prayer.

The minute you see the child, feel the child, you know that you can't help, that the only thing you can possibly do is to try and help the parents. You take this baby and rush to the unit going through the motion of resuscitation. You race to the hospital on a hopeless errand. You bring the child into the hospital so that they can sit the parents in a small private room painted in soothing colors and tell them that they did everything they could but it wasn't enough.

Your only goal in this is to make sure the parents don't remember their home as a place of death. Let the hospital hold the title of "where my child died." and let their home be a place of good memories.

PATTI PRANKS

For a period of time I had a partner named Patti. Patti is a wonderful person and one of the most compassionate people I've ever worked with. She can find empathy for every patient and treat them all with respect, but she was also compulsive about cleaning in the truck which isn't a bad thing, but it was fun to abuse her over.

The key to driving Patti crazy was to slightly mess things up. She couldn't handle it. She would have to straighten every little item. If I really wanted to send her into a tizzy I would lick the tips of my fingers and put a fingerprint, just one, on each and every window and clear cabinet door in the ambulance. It would cause her to stress, to no end, until she could get her Windex bottle and clean it.

Patti was also a smoker but one of the ones that are constantly trying to quit. She made the grave error one day of asking me to help her quit. I told her I would be happy to, but she would need to be prepared for some tough love. She asked what I meant by that. I picked up her pack of cigarettes and licked the tips to all of them. She went completely apoplectic and was hollering at me asking me if I was crazy. I just told her.....tough love.

My goal from that day on was to catch her sitting her cigarettes down where I could get to them. I kept a syringe filled with a foul liquid air freshener and if I got them I would inject a little in all the cigarettes. Later that day she would be smoking away and get a mouthful of nasty. She would again ask if I was mental. Tough love darling, just tough love.

EASTER BAKING

It's a holiday weekend. Easter weekend to be precise. Not too bad as working holidays go. There are a few more people out and about but the Easter bunny doesn't usually bring doom and gloom like some of the other holidays can.

We get a call for an 80 year old lady with a possible broken hand. We head to the location which is her residence and are greeted at the door by an eightyish lady. "Are you who we are here for?" I ask. She tells us no, that she is in the kitchen could we come see.

Before we get to the kitchen I can her a loud humming sound and as I turn the corner I see one lady leaning over the oldest electrical mixer I have ever seen. She is being consoled by a third elderly female. The lady at the mixer has one hand in the mixing bowl and on closer evaluation she has three fingers wound into the beaters. The humming sound I heard is the mixer still trying to fold her fingers into the batter.

I am told by the three ladies that for the last 40 years they have gotten together on the day before Easter and baked all the cakes and sweets for Easter Sunday. Our mangled mixer of the three was attempting to taste the batter as the machine was running and had gotten her fingers grabbed.

I unplugged the machine from the wall and the lady let out a sigh of relief and looked at her friends and asked "why didn't ya'll do that?" The guilty look on their faces answered that question. No one even thought of it.

NOT FIT FOR THE NEWS

During New Orleans most violent of times the number of shootings and killings were huge. It was not uncommon to have three or four shootings a night with double that on the weekends. It got so bad that the news crews were like hyenas. They would listen to their scanners and rush to the scene of the shootings to take video. That video was usually pictures of EMS trying to save someone's life.

At first it was neat to get filmed, then it just got annoying as they crowded you on the scene, or just show you scrambling on a call in a non-flattering way.

We devised a rather evil method for preventing them from filming us. Our solution was to use our training. A gunshot victim would be considered a trauma patient. A trauma patient is a naked patient. That's the rule you are taught during your training. You wouldn't want to miss another gunshot or other injury.

We would cut the clothes away from a patients privates and expose them to the cameraman. They would get pissed knowing they couldn't use the film. This is before everyone could use a PC and blur the screen. They took their raw video and had it on the air in hours.

It became a game for us and them. They trying to get video and us trying to do anything we could to make it worthless.

RECOVERY DIVE

My pager went off with a number and 9-1-1 behind it. It was Police dispatch calling me on my day off. Whatever it is it can't be good. I make the call and am informed that three people have drowned in Bayou Bienvenue.

The story is that a man was fishing with his two young girls, ages 10 and 6, on the south side of the bayou. The 6-year-old fell in and the 10-year-old jumped in to save her. Both kids are reported to have been able to swim but the current was too strong. A stranger, a woman on the north side of the bayou, saw the kids go in the water and dove in herself to save them. All three drowned as they were pulled down by the current.

I was a member of the rescue team for the Sheriff's office. The drownings took place literally on the dividing line between my parish and Orleans. So the team that was put together to recover the drowning victims was from multiple agencies. We had Louisiana Wildlife and Fisheries Agents that worked our area as well as members of the New Orleans Police Department's Dive Team.

We all met up to figure our plan out. We knew that this grim task was to recover the bodies and give the family some closure. There was six of us so we would dive in teams of three with one team acting as support of the other while they were under the water. I was on the first team dive.

Bayou Bienvenue is a salt water bayou that drains the neighboring swamp land with the tides. One unique characteristic it has is, on the falling tide as the water is leaving the marsh and heading for open water, it is also draining the run off from the 50 year old land fill.

Our plan is to break down the bottom of the bayou into grids and each search our areas. There was a lot of ground to cover. I geared up and rolled over the side of the boat into dark water. The bottom was only 15 feet deep but the water was so muddy that visibility was measured in inches not feet. It was like diving in a bowl of soup. It was brown but not uniform in color, the shades of brown fluctuate and all of some sudden large globs of what looks like oil would appear in front of your mask and strike the glass, then drift around your head.

I start my search in this dark world and have to use all my self-control to stay focused on my search. My imagination is doing its level best to get the best of me. I am diving 15-foot-deep in brown water with three corpses. Every Saturday morning monster movie I ever watched is running through my head.

We have agreed that each dive will last 30 minutes. If we haven't found anything, we will swap out with the other team. The only thing that I found on my first dive was a crab trap I snagged my flipper strap on. I, of course, thought I had been grabbed and nearly shit my wet suit.

Breaking the surface into the sunshine is startling but the grave nature of our task dampens down any elation I might have. The second team goes in to start their search. We check our gear. We try to stay away from the news cameras filming us. We hope the other teams finds them even though we would never admit it.

I go in for my second search. It's just as dark and just as scary. I move with my arms out to my side to cover as much ground as I can. As I move I slide into a rhythm and a way to focus and that's when I bump face to face with the dead woman. I panic. Against everything I've been trained, I launch myself straight up breaking the surface like a Sea World exhibit. I am hyperventilating and can't get my words out but it's obvious I've found one of them.

I go back down and using all my courage get hold of her and bring her to the surface. The boat team lowers a body bag into the water so we can put her inside without the indecency of dragging her body over the gunwale of the boat in clear view of camera people.

We get her to the shore and see it is the lady who tried to save the young girls. She has been in the water only 6 hour, but the shrimp and crabs have already taken their pound of flesh.

We dive for two more days. The 6 year old's body surfaces on the second day. It will be another week before a fisherman finds the last girl in the marsh.

After all was over all the divers ended up with rashes from the tidal flow from the land fill. Nothing like doing a grisly job and having the itches to prove it.

~~MORTAL COMBAT~~

The craziest holiday of the year to work the streets is New Year's Eve. Everyone wants to party and a good portion of those, take it too far. Every year there are foolish people that celebrate using firearms instead of fireworks or some other attempt at Darwin award fame. The amount of alcohol consumed and drugs used has a major effect on the trouble people get into.

It had been a fairly quiet New Year's Eve so far. So that means we were just normal busy not insane busy. We actually had found a sheltered spot at midnight to ring in the New Year without being in the open for possible falling bullets. We were scheduled to get off at 2am and we were in the final stretch. I was working with Frank and his brother Joe who for some strange reason had volunteered to ride along on this New Year's shift. Dispatch calls with one more call.

We are sent to meet the Fire Department's Fire boat at the Mississippi river dock. The call is that a man fell or jumped off the pier near the French Quarter in to the Mississippi. The fire boat was going to fish him out of the water and bring him to us.

Now the weather was in the mid-50s and beautiful but the water in the river was substantially lower in temperature. The average was in the forties and that kind of wet cold can sap the strength, then the life right out of a person, not to mention the fatigue of fighting the current while swimming.

As we headed to the dock we started placing IV bags up on the dash and pushing the hot air of the defroster over them to heat up the fluids. We pulled our blankets out and prepared for a severely chilled patient.

Once we arrive on scene we head down the gangway and meet the boat as it arrives. Our patient is a man in his late twenties. He is pale and his lips are blue. The fire guys have wrapped him in blankets to try and warm him up. The three of us with the Fire Departments help get him off the boat and into the back of our unit.

First thing is warm IV bags in both armpits, along with the blankets and something on his head to help prevent heat loss. Frank gets up front to start our trip to the emergency room. I strip off his wet clothes and are setting up the IV that I will start on him. So far thing are going typical. I have Joe sitting at the patients head while I am on his left side on the bench seat. I put the tourniquet on his arm and lean over to make the needle stick. The very instant that the needle breaks our patients skin we realize our assumptions about our patient are very wrong.

Our patient goes ballistic! He starts swinging his arms and trying to get up and out of the unit. He starts yelling and laughing, a high pitch maniacal laugh. Crap! Happy New Year...

Our plan has now changed. It is time to restrain this animal for their own safety, not to mention the safety of the medics, namely me. Our suspicions at the time, that were later verified, was that our patient didn't fall in the river. He was high as a kite on PCP and jumped in the water while in a delusional state. Now we had warmed him up, woke him up, and pissed him off. Did I mention we were trapped with him in a small metal box!

I begin the task of trying to strap down his arms with Joes help, but every time we would get one secured he breaks it free. He is kicking and thrashing his head. I finally realize a heightened degree of violence may be needed.

I spin around and do my best WWE move and flop my ass down on my patient's chest and abdomen. Whoooosh!!! As all the air leaves his lungs. I'm yelling at him to stay still. I'm yelling at Joe to hold him down. I'm yelling at Frank to drive faster. Sooo, typical night for me.....

I've switched my radio to the medical control channel and tell them I'm coming with this whirling dervish. They can hear the crazy laughter and then screams in the background. I am told security will meet me on the hospital ramp.

After knocking the wind out of him I have a few seconds to secure his arms again. I am trying to get a strap across his chest and am leaning my right arm across his body to his right side. I was not paying close enough attention, because I had let my forearm get too close to his mouth and he snapped at me catching the hairs on my arm.

Now here is where I take a break from our story and discuss the fact that in most situations you would not want to cause any damage to a patient, especially any visible damage, like facial impacts. Joe my third rider is such a rookie that he is watching me and keying off me for what he deems as okay to do in this PCP rodeo.

With the hairs pulled out of my arm I rear back and give him a jab in the nose to make sure he understands that biting is off the table. Joe sees this action and believes that I have given the signal indicating the gloves are off and this is now a free for all. Joe rears back and starts repeatedly punching this guy in the head and face pow! Pow! Pow! POW! Crap, double crap. I have my hands full trying to hold him down (yes I was holding him as Joe beat him.) all I can do is yell. "NOT THE FACE!" "NOT THE FACE!"

My words finally get through to Joe after a plethora of hammer strikes and he stops. I am pretty sure that all this did was piss our patient off more. He has again broken an arm free is kicking his legs and thrashing about. I hop straight up in the air and give him a couple of body bounces. I radio the hospital that we are on final approach and that I'm having to ride him like a bull to control him and my 8 seconds were up ages ago. Frank is enjoying my suffering as I can hear him laughing from the front of the truck at Joe and I.

We turn the final corner and roll up the ramp. I feel the brakes engage and the truck stop. Both the rear doors fly open at once and Brian, one of the Paramedics from another truck is standing there. He puts both of his arms up in the classic herculean pose and yells "MORTAL COMBAT!!" and dives in the truck directly on top of me and the patient.

~~BLIND MAN'S BLUFF~~ ~~~~~~~~~~~~~~~~~~~~~~~

For some reason, when you're trained as a medic, people think you suddenly have the knowledge to deal with mental illness. Yes it is an illness but usually not the kind a medic is trained for. Not to the degree that an expert in it would be, but it always seems that these calls come your way.

I was working in a sprint car which means I was by myself and in a car running to calls first and evaluating them. I would then determine if a full crew and unit was needed and could get started on the patient care and the report.

I was given a call for a psych patient. This patient called us fairly frequently. He would call when he was depressed or when he and his parents would fight. He was in his 30s and had suffered a traumatic injury ten years prior and had lost his sight. His sanity had slipped soon after.

I pulled up to the house and walked to the front door, it's a glass storm door. It's very bright outside so I couldn't see into the house. I knocked and I heard Lee, our patient, yell. "Come in." I opened the door and stepped in. It's very dim in the living room so it took a second for my eyes to adjust.

Once I could see again I saw Lee sitting on the sofa and pointing what looks like a .22 Cal target pistol at me. Oh crap! "Lee, it's alright man I'm here to help, put the gun down." The more I talked it seemed like he was honing in on my voice and the pistol's aim improved.

He begun to say how depressed he was and how he wanted to die and how we never listened and at the moment he is completely correct, since all I could do was focus on the barrel of that pistol.

I eased my way over to the right and turned my handheld radio off. I figured as long as he was rambling on and I didn't have the barrel pointed at my chest we were making progress.

I damn near shit my pants when my pager went off. He swung the gun and immediately got a bead on me. Son of a bitch....I turned off the pager, tried not to hyperventilate and eased back in the other direction.

This went on for what felt like hours but couldn't have been more than 4 or 5 minutes. I knew the crew coming to the scene would be wondering why I wasn't answering the radio and get concerned. I hope they sped up.

I heard the brakes on the back up unit out front. Lee heard them too, because I could see him moving his head, listening towards the door and still talking to me. I continued to make my way around the room and now I've gotten close to him.

Sometimes stupidity in others can benefit you. In this case the medic in the unit sent to assist me, instead of showing caution, since I was off the air, walked right up to the door pulled it open and exclaimed "Hey fucker, you're not answering your radio!" Lee immediately took a bead on her. I took this moment to grab for the gun and wrestle it out of Lee's grip. The medic that barged in had obviously not expected to find a gun pointed at her by a blind man, since she promptly pissed herself. That's what happens when you call me fucker and do stupid things.

THAT SHIT WILL STOP

A program that we had at the city was for the new emergency docs to come and work in the field and ride along with the Supervisors. They would show up on scenes and have the opportunity to see the cases as we saw them and give us medical orders right there. This was designed to give them a better idea of our world and for us all to build a good rapport with them.

We get the call for a double shooting. The caller said two guys shot in a car. We head that way and Darrell the Supervisor lets us know that he and the doctor were also responding.

My partner and I get to the scene first and walk over to the car, and sure enough there are two guys in the front seat of the car. The driver has a point blank gunshot to the face. A large portion of his head is in the backseat. He is obviously very dead. The passenger has a gunshot through the temple. His head is leaning on his chest and there is gray matter in his lap.

I go around to the passenger side of the car and lift that patients head up just as doc and Darrell walk up. I lift his head and he makes a motion that we call fish breathing. He opens his mouth and makes the O like motion but the diaphragm doesn't work so no air moves. Doc sees this and blurts out "He's breathing!!" Darrell looks right at doc and with the firmest tone possible he says, "Oh but no that shit will stop!"

ENTREPRENEURIAL SPIRIT

We often cruised in and around the French Quarter when it was slow. It's always fun to people watch. To see the tourists enjoying the city, its history and festivities, but some people are not streetwise and can have advantage taken of them.

As we were cruising one day we saw an obvious tourist couple walking away from the French Quarter and the recognizable touristy spots. They were headed directly toward one of the city's housing projects. A very poor choice of places to visit. It is high on excitement but low on historical value.

We pull up next to them and say hello and ask them where they were going. They hand me a map and say they were following a free walking tour that some kids had given them. Being from small town Middle America, these folks thought that giving out free tours was a mighty nice thing for these young men to do. I look at the map and it shows a path from the French Quarter directly through the housing project.....hmmmmm....Me smells a rat!

We have the couple jump in the unit with us and cruise down the path on their flyer. Sure enough there is a group of very predatory looking local urban youths loitering on a porch in the shadows. We point them out to our passengers and explain that the only historical thing along their route may have been them. We take them back to a safe area and send them on their merry way and grab the first NOPD cop we can find. We go with him to where the tourists told us they got the flyer, and there standing in the middle of Bourbon St. are two young (early teens) boys passing out flyers from a stack.

The Police scoop them up and confiscate their flyers. The police informed us later that the kids were getting paid a percentage of the loot gained from the people they routed into danger. The local Kinko's was asked to please look a little closer at the flyer orders in the future.

~~VANITY~~

Being vane is something everyone at one point or another has dealt with personally in their life. Whether it is as a teenager fighting the hormones of youth or as an adult dealing with body image issues. It can be a problem and sometimes it can lead down a very dark road.

The call was a welfare check on a possible suicide. The person that called the police said that one of their friends and former co-worker had called her to tell her goodbye. He told her he was going to take his life.

We get to the residents and the front door is unlocked. As we search the house we find the bathroom is the only door that we can't access. We knock we call his name and there is no answer. I'm given the go ahead to finesse the lock on the bathroom, so we can get inside and it takes only a minute to gain access.

As I swing open the door I am shocked by the scene. The person we were sent to check on is lying in the tub with his hands resting on the sides as if he is relaxing. His skin is porcelain white. He had laid towels down underneath himself and they are soaked in his blood. His feet are crossed at the ankles and kicked up by the faucet. He looked peaceful but that is deceiving since I can also see the bloody foot prints on the tub wall where he thrashed around in pain and fear of the end. As his blood loss got more profound, he felt euphoric and took up this peaceful pose.

His method was sound. Sitting on the lid of the toilet was a glass, half full, of vodka. The ice in the glass hadn't melted yet. He had used a razor blade cutting from his wrist to his elbow on the inside of his left arm first. He only made it 8 inches on the right arm, but it, mixed with the vodka, was more than enough to empty his body of blood.

    His note was on the vanity. He had killed himself in the bathroom to prevent making a mess for his family. He said that his face had been scarred in an accident a year prior and he could not live with being disfigured any longer.

    I looked deeply at this poor soul and searched his face. I could not find the scar that so troubled him and ultimately caused him to take his life.

HEAVY

There seems to be an unwritten formula when it comes to patients that need to be carried. It goes something like this. The further back in a house or higher up in floors, the heavier the patient will be. I think it's an inverse square root thing.

It's the call you don't want to hear. Patient short of breath, on the third floor, in the back of the apartment.......by the way she weighs in at 600 lbs. Crapola!

My partner John and I get on the scene and climb up to the apartment. We find our patient in a bedroom in the back as dispatch had previously warned us. There was **NO** exaggeration in her weight. She is six bills if she is a pound. She is sitting on the edge of her bed and is in obvious severe distress. Her 15 year old daughter is with her. The daughter is 300 lbs. and well on her way to matching her mother in gravitational pull. The daughter tells us that her mother hasn't been out of the house in six years and she hasn't been off the third floor in the last two!

First things first. We call the Fire Department and ask to get some help sent our way. I have no idea how we are going to get her out of here yet. My brain is running on overtime trying to treat her medical needs and formulate an engineering plan that will allow us to get her out of this place without removing a wall.

We decided we will try and get her on a device called a stair chair. It's exactly what it sounds like it's a chair with wheels that is designed to be lowered down the steps. There is only one problem. It's only rated for 400 lbs. We can only hope it is over engineered for the extra weight since it's the best chance we have.

We need the patient to help us slide from the bed to the stair chair. We do all we can to assist her as she moves but the strain on her system is so bad at this point that it's like she is climbing Mount Everest her body can't take the strain and her heart stops.

We lower her as best we can to the ground. Things have just gotten exponentially more difficult. Fire department guys are on the scene now to help and we need to get her out of the house as quickly as possible all the while attempting some form of CPR.

Now I consider myself a pretty strong guy. I work out I lift weights, but that's steel plates. A human body doesn't stay rigid it wants to shift and roll and the bigger a person is the harder it becomes. There is no hand hold to help lift.

We decide that we are going to tie a rope around her chest and lower her down the stairs. One of us will basically ride her down like a sled so we can perform CPR. We thought about carrying her but even if we could lift her she is wider than the stairwell. None of the boards we have would hold her and maybe if we had the time to formulate a plan we could come up with a better idea but time is the one thing that she doesn't have. The odds we could save her to start with were extremely thin and that got anorexic the more time that passes.

We began to descend the first set of stairs. Three fireman and a medic on the rope, another medic on the patient. It is about as absurd a sight as could ever be imagined. We strain and lower and sweat and groan as we ease her down the stairs. It is not a graceful action for her or us.

We make the second floor landing and take a few minutes to reset our ropes, continue what medical care we can, and catch our breath before the next flight.

The next flight goes very much the same as the last. Her body rubs both walls on the way down her arms continually get tangled as she moves down. It is an indignity that I wish we could spare her, but our job is to save people if we can and the fact that she died in front of us means we have an obligation to do everything we can to get her back.

We make it to the first floor and out on to the porch. We suddenly see another hurdle in our way. First, our stretcher is not rated for her weight. Second, she is at least three times as wide as the stretcher. We decide on the fly to leave the stretcher out of the truck. The fire department can carry it for us. We back the truck up to the porch and slide her on to the floor of the unit. She fills the area completely. I have her on the cardiac monitor and notice that as we do normal CPR we are getting almost nothing to indicate we are being effective. I push harder and harder and still see no affect.

In what I have come too classified as Bruce Lee CPR, I pull back my right hand and make a first. I throw a punch using all my weight putting my hips in to the thrust and let out a "KIA!" and impact directly over her heart. I make a mental note to thank my Sensei because the monitor showed success. I keep this up left, right, left, right, until I need to call the hospital. We are moving that way and I will need their help. I don't have a stretcher nor is there anyway on this planet that John and I could get her out of here on our own.

I switch CPR techniques to knee CPR, using my body weight to compress the chest. It isn't as effective as Bruce Lee CPR, but it will do for the few seconds of the phone call. I call the hospital and give them the run down. I have a 600 pound cardiac arrest patient. We witnessed her arrest and we are coming to you. We will be there in 3 minutes. We need you to bring a big boy stretcher (An actual thing I swear.) out to the ramp so we can get her out the truck. The person on the other end of the phone says "ah huh, sure." and hangs up. Well that was rude.

We finish our transport and pull onto the ramp and ....crickets. No one outside. No stretcher!?! No help! Well this isn't good.

My partner runs in and calls for some assistance. They start saying they thought it was a practical joke, so they ignored the call. Once they realize we were serious, the mad scrambling begins.

We finally get enough help to muscle our patient out of the truck and onto the big boy stretcher. Then it's a sprint into the hospital. The E.R. staff works very hard to save her but in the end it just wasn't enough. Her heart was no longer strong enough to handle the stress of her size and nothing we did could change that.

~~BITE~~ ME

Sometimes you try and do a good deed, and it turns around and bites you in the ass. I unfortunately had a situation like this that was all too literal.

We got a call for a guy sprayed with mace. NOPD had subdued him and had him in custody. We met them on the scene and found our patient. He was rude and belligerent and, in general, an asshole to us, as we flushed his eyes and wiped his face of the residual spray. We completed our report and left the scene, headed to our next call. Usually I would never give him another thought, but fate had something different in mind.

About an hour later I was sitting on the tailgate of my ambulance, writing a report as it seems I was always doing. Coming up the ramp is the NOPD officer we had talked to earlier and he was pushing a Charity Hospital Wheelchair with my mace guy handcuffed to it. It seems he had fought them, again, and he had been maced, again, so they needed to get him evaluated before the jail would accept him.

As I am talking to the officer the lunatic in the wheelchair begins thrashing from side to side. He throws himself so violently that he tips over the wheelchair and since he is handcuffed to it, he is now hanging out of it on the ground.

This is where I made my error. I felt bad for the Officer, and stepped up to help right the wheelchair. As I had my arm across his body, to gain leverage on the chair; the mace faced lunatic bit me, and I don't mean a little bite. I mean a pit bull latch on to my forearm.

Now over my years I have been beaten on, kicked, and on at least one occasion stabbed. I have been shot at and missed and shit at and hit, but something about this guy sinking his teeth into my flesh made me lose my mind.....

    As soon as he clamped down on my left arm I started hammering him in the face with my right fist. I beat him until he let go, then I beat him until he was unconscious. I'm pretty sure I beat all the teeth out of his head. The NOPD Officer was torn between apologizing for the guy biting me and freaked over having to explain the beaten and handcuffed guy in his wheelchair.

    I made the report on the bite on me, to cover me for my assault on him, and explain things for the poor cop. I also had to get medical care for the chunk bitten out of me. In the end the guy went to jail...... on a liquid diet.

RESCUING ROSE

I rode out hurricane Katrina with my wife at her work. She was the transportation Manager for a major uptown hospital, and I was able to put our personal vehicles high up in a parking garage. She was also able to bring our pets to stay with us. Mostly it was the fact that she was pregnant with our son and I wanted to be close.

As the storm assaulted the hospital, we watched the water rise and threaten. We had the power go out but we weathered it well. In the hours after the storm passed we watched the waters recede. We thought that the worst was behind us.

We talked and felt that she would have to stay the night and be allowed to head home the next day. It was decided I would take our dogs home, get into uniform and go to work. I was working with the U.S. Marshall's Service on the fugitive recovery task force. I knew they would be part of any rescue work and wanted to help.

I loaded up my unit and drove right out of the parking garage on mostly dry streets and headed home. There was of course downed trees and damaged buildings and signs but at the time I thought we had dodged a bullet.

I couldn't have been more wrong.

By the time I talked to my wife that night the water had come back up and was eight foot deep in front of the hospital. We didn't know it at the time but this was the result of the levees failing and the onslaught of water storming through the city.

I went to work and for the next two days I worked as a medic, a cop, a food server and whatever else needed doing. At night I was pulling carpet from my home that water had risen in and talking to my wife when I could, hearing how it was getting worse at the hospital.

You see, sometime in the hours after I had left her the levees had failed. This brought eight foot of water right back to the doors of the hospital. Trapping everyone inside.

She told me how the basement had flooded and the generator was underwater. The kitchen had been in the basement so it was underwater. She was holding up but I knew she wanted out. She was in a building that was like a deserted island in deep water.

The morning of the third day with phone calls becoming more and more difficult to get through my wife was able to get a phone call out to me. She was frantic. She said it was really bad and she needed to get out. She said "Please come get me!" I knew I would do whatever it took to get her out safety.

I was already in my tactical gear. My bullet proof vest, gun belt and my rifle. I had worked a lot of extra hours to get my rifle. It was a gorgeous Rock River Arms M-4 with all the bells and whistles. It had been a serious point of contention since I had gotten it between my wife and I. She just did not understand why I needed it. I got in my unit and headed to her. I had no plan or idea just the goal that I would get her to safety and I was determined to stop at nothing to succeed.

I crossed the Mississippi River Bridge and got on Tchoupitoulas St. which ran along the Mississippi river. I knew it was some of the highest ground in the city and was most likely dry. I made it to Napoleon Ave which the hospital was on and headed north. I got as far as St Charles Ave. This is where I found the beginning of the water and a sea of people as well.

The first thing I come across as I step out of my car is a National guardsman in fatigues all by himself. He has his M-16 and no magazine in it. I ask him what he was doing. He tells me that his Captain dropped him off here to guard the corner but gave him no further instructions, nor any ammunition. I pulled a full magazine from my vest and gave it to him. He was very thankful and as I told him what I was trying to do. He told me that there was an airboat that was shuttling a few people from the area. I told him to be safe and headed out.

I walked into the water and sure enough an old guy with a bayou accent was on an airboat that was tied up to a stop sign. I stepped up and did the most illegal thing I have ever done. I lifted my rifle signaling him my intentions without actually pointing it at him. I told him I'm taking your boat. I need to get my wife. Without a word he got out. I climbed up into the seat.

Now I have driven boats all my life, but this thing had 2 sticks and no wheel. I stepped back down where the old man was standing with his hands in his pockets and I looked right at him and told him "I'm taking you too." The old man laughed at me and got in the boat and asked "Where we goin Cap?"

I stood at the bow of the boat rifle at the ready and guided him to the hospital. I was stunned to be boating over the streets I had drove over just days earlier. We skidded over the roofs of cars sunken in the depths of the road and watched as we dodged stop signs and wove a path through the water and debris.

We made the turn to the emergency room entrance. It was on the second floor and barely out of the water. The E.R. ramp was crowded with people everyone wanted out and they were essentially trapped. This place that had been a place of refuge was now a prison. Powerless, overheated and running out of food and water.

	I see my wife on the ramp and I am elated. I really had no clue whether I was going to be able to get to her. I signal her over to the boat where my new best friend and I tie up. The last thing I want to do is get out of my appropriated boat and get left. She comes over and we hug but there will be time for that later. She asks if we can take some of her employees with us and I can't refuse. The more people sharing in my felony the better.

	I signal my hostage/ pilot/ accomplice and we head back toward St. Charles and dry land. We offload my rescued crew and I thank the old guy and apologize for taking him hostage. He says he has a wife to and not to worry about it. I'll always be thankful to him.

	As we get to my unit and the sea of people surrounding it, I have to move people away with the help of the National Guardsman and load everyone up. There are a lot of desperate people and I promise to do what I can to help them. The National Guardsman is kind enough to helps keep the crowd back as we prepare to leave. I hand him some more ammo and some snacks and wish him luck. I put the car in gear and head toward home. My wife looks at the rifle that I have in the front seat with us and she tells me. "I will never say another word about that thing again in my life."

ANIMAL CONTROL

When you're on a call there are all sorts of things that get in the way. There's the layout of the house, the furniture, nosey neighbors and so many other things but what has caused more havoc on calls for me have been dogs. It's because of the love they have for their owners most of the time that causes them to get in the way and underfoot. Not all of my partners have had the same love for our four legged friends as I do causing odd results.

Our patient is a nice enough older lady having chest pains. Her pet is a maniacal and neurotic Chihuahua named Eddie. Eddie has been yipping and yapping since we set foot in the house. My partner, who will remain nameless to protect their identity, must have a special smell because Eddie has not stopped snapping and nipping at his pants leg. He keeps pushing the dog away with his leg and Eddie charges back to latch on to a pant leg and shake it for all he's worth. Eddie's owner just keeps saying "Eddie stop being rude. He really is kind and friendly." My partner mumbles something that sounded like "my ass." under his breath.

By now I am fairly amused at the whole affair and can't help but make it worse. I am setting up the IV for our patient and I squirt Eddie with the fluid as I bleed the line. Eddie is so focused on my partner he is sure he is the culprit and amps up his attack. Now Eddies pissed, my partner is none too happy. I'm having a ball.

We are packaging our patient on the stretcher and have her on oxygen, the cardiac monitor and have her IV started. My partner has had his fill of Eddie and I can see the frustration.

I believe that Eddie had finally taken it one step too far when he mauled my partner's shoe-strings and retaliation was fast approaching.

Now at the time we had a Lifepak 5 cardiac monitor. It had an interesting setting on the defibrillator. You could run a test defib at 5 joules instead of upwards of 300 joules.

All of a sudden I hear the monitor charging, that high pitch windup is unmistakable. I look over at the evil grin forming on my partners face. He was kneeling next to the stretcher and just casually turned and hit the discharge buttons.

Eddies ass levitates off the ground like he was possessed. He lets out a squeal that would pierce your ears and seems to be running before his little feet hit the ground. He looked like a scene out of a Loony Tunes cartoon.

Eddies Owner asks what happened. My partner says in a dead pan voice "Eddie was shocked that we hadn't left for the hospital yet and was insisting that we go." I was the one who was shocked when our patient said. "Eddie is always putting me first. Isn't that sweet of him?"

MACHETE MAN

One of the stranger combinations that I have been involved in here in Louisiana is as a medic for a Sheriff's office. We carried guns, wore police style uniforms and were certified as cops but our primary job was responding to emergency medical calls.

One of the things that we also did was committals for psychiatric observation. One of our units had gone out on one just a few blocks from where I was stationed. I was again in a sprint car so when I heard them get on scene I thought I'd cruise in that direction in case they needed anything.

As I'm headed in that direction I hear the unit on the scene whispering into the radio. They say they are in the house with the patient's mother and the guy they are there to pick up is in the backyard. The problem is he is ranting and raving talking to unseen creatures and wielding a 3 foot machete.

I am only a block away so I let them know I'm coming. They tell me they will meet me out front when I get there, so we can get a game plan together.

I pull to the front of the house and hit my brakes. They let out a chatter and squeak that is ear shattering. So much for a stealthy entrance. I step out of the car and I'm standing on the curb when machete man comes out of the back yard.

He is big. Six two, six three or so, well built and bat shit fucking crazy. His eyes are black and dilated so that they look, as said by Capt. Quin, like dolls eyes. His entire demeanor says don't fuck with me I'm not right. That and the fact that he has a huge machete raised in his hand makes me want to heed the warning but damned if I don't have a job to do.

He is walking not running towards me with the machete raised. There is no doubt he is intending to do me harm. I draw my gun and time slows down. I am yelling for him to stop and drop the weapon but my voice sounds far away. The little voice in my head is repeating, stop dude please stop. I don't want to shoot you.

He keeps coming and I am tightening down on the trigger. I have drawn a mental line on the lawn in front of me. If he crosses that spot I will have no choice but to shoot him.

One step closer. He is less than a foot from the point of no return. There is tension on the trigger and only a hairs pull from firing.

At the moment that I commit to my task and prepare to shoot, him he suddenly stops. He turns the flat side of the machete towards himself and starts hitting himself with the broadside of the blade. He is screaming about being on fire as he crumbles to the lawn. The other crew has come out the front door as this was going on and we secure him and take away the machete.

I will never know what made him stop. I have no problem doing what must be done, but I am grateful that this obviously troubled man will not be one of the things that keep me up at night.

HAROLD

Some people leave a bigger mark in your life than others and Harold was that kind of person. He was small in stature and large in personality. Harold was one of our day shift rescue guys but he was so much more. He was 20 years older than most of us so he had that big brother, big uncle vibe, always friendly and always willing to help. We had a large flock of pigeons that lived in the truck bay and Harold took the time to feed them every day where most others would have ignored them at best. He was also the guy you wanted backing you up on a scene. The man had ice water in his veins. You knew things were all right when he was around.

I was just finishing my night shift on a Saturday morning and crews were coming in to work Lollapalooza. I got on my Harley to head out and as I was leaving Harold was coming in. He was a big motorcycle fan and gave me a big smile and a double thumbs up. I had no clue that he was suffering with chest pains already and just wasn't sharing this information with anyone.

Several hours later after dropping a patient off at the emergency room his partner persuaded him to seek care. They diagnosed with a major heart attack. I came back to work that night to learn that he was in the hospital and it didn't look good.

My partner and I for the night got asked to handle a special transfer. They wanted us to transfer Harold from the Charity hospital where he had been treated earlier that day, to Tulane hospital a few blocks away so that the cardiologist there could handle his care.

As we waited in the hallway of the Cardiac Care Unit the frenzy erupts that means only one thing a Cardiac Arrest. Harold had coded. We were right there and there was nothing we could do to help. We were observers in what was normally the game we played. It's a battle that is like rolling back time. Death has already arrived and you try and fight it, to back it down if only for a while.

Harold lost the battle that night and no amount of fighting from him or the valiant staff could turn the tide. We had all lost a hero.

How do you celebrate the life of someone you worked with in the trenches? Someone that helped you keep death at bay for hundreds of people but has finally lost their battle. You don't have to do anything but let the people come and honor him. It will show in those that his life impacted and made a difference.

The services would be a large affair. The family of medics fire fighters and police always stand together to salute their own in their final rides. There would be representatives from every service in the region a procession of ambulances, fire trucks and police cars that would be miles long. It is a testament to the love we had for him to see so many pay their respects.

Public service has a tradition that is unique due to the nature of our jobs. It is called Last Call. Harold's Unit, 6232, is draped with banners of mourning and driven with lights but no sirens. As the procession gets close to our EMS station, Dispatch calls for 6232 over the air.

Dispatch gives his unit its last call.

"6232, 6232 respond to 1700 Moss St. (the EMS station) Signal 'Last Call' Code 2."

Charlie Brown a longtime friend of Harold's and the senior rescue person stands in to answer the call.

"6232, 10-4, enroute from 3827 Canal St. (The funeral home)"

"10-4, 6232"

"6232" Charlie has to stop, he is so choked up, "6232 10-97, 10-7 9-29-97"

The quaver in Charlie's voice is felt and shared by everyone on the air. Marking him 10-7 'completely out of service' and the date of his death is a sting felt in the heart.

I myself am sobbing and the tears poor down my face. There isn't a dry eye in the unit with me.

Dispatch acknowledges that he is out of service and retires him.

AS we proceed to the cemetery I clearly remember a former co-worker and follow Paramedic that now works for the State Police standing on the side of the road as we pass. He is at rigid attention and holding a knife sharp salute, but I can clearly see the tears rolling from under his aviator sunglasses.

I often think of Harold and how he affected me in my growth in EMS. How he was always an ear to listen and a friend to talk with. He would always take the time to show a rookie the ropes. I have always tried to be the kind of mentor to others that Harold was to me. It's a legacy that should always be passed on.

~~DOUBLE YELLOWS~~

Before there were two bridges crossing the Mississippi River in New Orleans, traffic traveled in both directions on the same bridge. Instead of having a barricade between them they had an empty lane that was bordered on both sides by double yellow lines.

It was a zone that emergency vehicles could run with lights and sirens to expedite crossing the river. The catch is you needed to call and get permission to enter the double yellows. You had to make sure no one was coming from the other direction.

We were downtown which is the east bank of the river and had just received an emergency call on the Westbank. We turn on the lights and sirens and off we go. We're already heading up the on ramp for the bridge as we call dispatch to get permission to enter the double yellow. They give us the okay right away so this should be fun!

It's a rush to speed down this lane with traffic on both sides of you but it's not without its dangers. As we are racing toward the peak of the bridge dispatch suddenly tells us we are not clear! They are very excited. I take my foot off the throttle and coast for a second as we try to sort this out.

Before we can get a handle on things a police car tops the bridge and we are steaming head on with each other. We both lock up our brakes. There is nowhere to go. Left is into oncoming traffic. Right is into crowded westbound lanes. The distance Narrows as we slide three tons worth of ambulance forward. The nose of the police car is scraping the ground. Crap this is going to be hurt!

Two inches, that's the gap between our vehicles when we come to a stop. Just two inches. No damage to the vehicles but I'm pretty sure I needed a new pair of shorts.

ROCK AND ROLL DETAIL

Details are extra jobs you can do to make more money outside of your regular shifts. These vary from things like working the side lines for high school football games, working foot races, maybe even manning a medical tent at a festival of some sort, but the best detail I ever worked was a concert. A very particular concert.

I was asked if I would work a detail for a concert in City Park. Whose playing I ask? The Ramones and Pearl Jam. Are you fucking with me? Of course I'll work it.

The concert was held at Tad Gormley Stadium. It was home of the US Track and Field Olympic Trials in 1992. It holds 26,500 people in the seats but this concert would not just fill the seats. It was expected to have 42,000 people in attendance.

The reasons they needed medics there was pretty obvious. Anytime you put that many people in one place partying, someone will need medical attention, probably a bunch of someones. Not to mention it was the law that they had to have so many medics per 1000 people or something like that.

So we found ourselves on site on a Saturday morning hours before the show. We set up a medical tent and had meetings on how we would get people in and out of the crowd.

I got very lucky since Raymond and I were the biggest guys we were given the plum job of working the edges of the stage. Our job would be to pull anyone in the very front rows out and treat them since getting into that crowd would be a nightmare.

Once we were all ready the only thing left to do was wait. It was still several hours before the show and the people were just trickling in. They had a hospitality tent set up with food and drinks and we were told to feel free to get something when we had the chance. I headed over to eat, figuring I wouldn't get a chance once the show started.

I, for the life of me, couldn't tell you what I ate because as I was sitting there by myself eating who sits down across from me but Joey Ramone. I mean Joey 'Friggin' Ramone!! He and the band sat at the table and just started bullshiting with me. Joey was so cool and down to earth, they all were. I was a fan already, but after meeting him and the band, I was hooked.

In contrast Eddie Vedder and the band were pretty reclusive. They weren't rude or anything they just stayed in their trailer, except to catch part of the Ramones show. It's as if they needed to psych themselves up for their own time on stage.

The lights dim and I'm standing at the top of the stairs, stage right, just as the band comes up and takes the run up and storms onto the dais. The lights come up and they charge right into the song 'Animal'. The crowd rushes the stage.

The energy is palpable. It is amazing. This is my first encounter on this side of a crowd this big and I can completely understand how powerful a performer feels in front of the crowd. I was just the medic in the wings and I was pumped up off the charts.

I can see Raymond across the stage and all we can do is share a shit eating grin with each other. When you look out on the sea of people and witness two giant mosh pits. You see people crowd surfing and you think, damn they are paying me to be here. All you could do is smile and laugh at the absurdity of it all.

The strongest memory of the show was standing there as the band starts into 'Even Flow' and I am keying up the radio on a spare channel so dispatch and all the street units can hear. It was exhilarating.

~~PARKING TICKET~~

Parking in the city of New Orleans, and the French Quarter in particular, can be a pain in the ass. Granted it's not New York but what we gain in space to park we make up for with Meter Nazis of the first order. New Orleans has a Private company that writes and collects fees for parking violations so they epitomize the quota seekers we all fear and despise.

An Ambulance in the French Quarter is its own sort of problem. The streets were built in the early 1700s for horse drawn carriage not for modern vehicles and especially for huge box style ambulances.

You surely can't park one in a normal spot, if you could even find one. It is not uncommon when getting calls in the Quarter to double park in front of the location and leave the lights on while you go in and handle the call.

On this day we are responding to a chest pain at one of the big tourist restaurants in the French Quarter. We double park and go take care of business.

We come out with our patient and start loading them in the truck. I head to the driver's door to get this patient to the hospital and what do I find but a meter maid standing in front of my unit. She is writing us a parking ticket. I first try reason.

Yes. I know that was foolish of me.

As I tell her we are an emergency vehicle on a call she stares at me as if I am speaking in tongues. I next threaten to call the Police, she continues to just stare at me never uttering a word.

Later I learn that the company that manages the tickets gets one dollar for every ticket written no matter if they are thrown away or paid. It's a straight up racket.

I finally resort to the one thing I'm good at.....brute force. I get in the truck put it in gear and pull forward until she is forced to dive out of the way. I couldn't help but laugh as the crowd gave me a round of applause.

COUSINS

Family. Arguably, the most important thing in life. My cousin Richie and I were not especially close, but like family in the south, when we did cross paths, we had that easy way of sliding back in to conversation and being comfortable with each other. We had grown up in and out of each other's lives. We played little league together. We saw each other at all the family gatherings.

After I left for the Army and then returned to the police department our contacts were very sparse. He had gotten in some trouble with the law when I was gone and we just hadn't crossed paths. I would have never dreamed that our next meeting would be such a tragic event.

I received a call for a man not breathing so we rolled to the address. As I arrived two things struck me immediately. First I recognized the house and second one of my uncles were standing on the porch. I immediately had a sinking dread in my stomach and my hands got clammy. I tasted that coppery taste in my mouth.

I got out and approached and my uncle looks pale and very shaken. He says, "It's Richie. He's in the bathroom." I head in the house with no gear. My brain is on autopilot. I walk back to the bathroom door and enter.

Richie is sitting on the closed toilet lid, slumped over against the sink. He has a set up kit for injection on the sink edge and a tourniquet around his arm. The needle is still hanging from the inside bend of his elbow. He has been dead for many hours. This is not a medical scene, there is nothing I can do.

I step out to confirm for my uncle what he already knows. I have a lump in my throat that I have to keep swallowing along with taking a deep breath to keep a firm grip on my professional composure.

I make the call to the hospital to confirm his death and to get things rolling with the coroner. Richie is only in his twenties. He will have to go to the coroner's office for an autopsy.

I have to call my mother and grandmother to tell them. I want to hesitate and take the coward's way out. If I wait long enough someone else will tell them but that's not the right thing to do. It is gut wrenching to get on the phone and tell them. It's worse than the thought of his death alone. Feeling their pain is much more traumatic than living with my own. It's a task I have had to do many times, and despise it more each time.

My final task I perform for my cousin is that I have to take him to the morgue. My partner and others offer to handle this without me, but I couldn't allow that. First, I owe it to my cousin to finish what I started and second, I owe it to my partner to be there. I need to be strong and handle my job. We package him up and make the trip. I leave him with a touch through the plastic of the body bag and a quick prayer. The prayer isn't for him. Any bed that he made, cannot be changed now. The prayer is for all his family and friends that will have to endure the grief and pain of the loss of one so young by such a distressing means.

DOUG'S IMPERIAL LOUNGE

Saturday nights the world over are known for being a time to throw down and party wherever you are, and in a city like New Orleans party time is always taken to the next level. Sometimes, there is a combination of forces that push the fun over the top even for the Big Easy.

This story is about just such a Saturday night. The forces of nature that collided that night were the combination of Saturday night, the closing of shrimping season, and everyone in the shrimping fleet celebrating at Doug's Imperial Lounge. Doug's was a truly high class joint (Read with a high degree of sarcasm). It was strategically located, being that it was connected to the Imperial Lanes bowling alley, for the most discerning of customer.

Now this occurred in the suburbs of New Orleans in a Parish (County for those of you not in Louisiana) that bordered Orleans Parish. The police force had a total of six, one-man patrol cars for the entire Parish, plus our two man rescue unit and a night dispatcher. This was for 75,000 residents.

It's after midnight and dispatch puts out a call to a patrol unit of a fight at Doug's. No one is surprised to hear this on a Saturday night. A second unit says they will back them up. As the rescue unit I didn't think much of this as we were required to stay free for "real" emergencies.

Those first units put themselves on scene. It didn't take long to hear one of the units call a 10-55 which is an Officer needs assistance call. There was four remaining units, one of them was tied up on a call but the other three put themselves enroute to back up the ones needing assistance. The on scene units were saying it was a big through down.

The next two units got on the scene and again, within minutes, they called for backup. There is only one unit left free so I grab my partner and we head toward the bar.

We run lights and sirens and beat the last unit to the scene. The parking lot is empty of people but packed with cars including four empty police cruisers. We head to the door and we can hear the heavy percussion of the music through the walls.

As we open the door we are struck, I mean physically struck, by a flying table. Yes, a fucking table came flying out the door at us. After dodging the table we rush into the fray and find ourselves in the middle of a full out bar brawl. It looks like an old west movie scene.

There is no telling who is a good guy or who is a bad guy. All the cops are still close to the entrance so we start grabbing anyone close to the doors and dragging them out.

The first group I dive into I grab one guy in an arm bar and while attempting to turn him around I get punched in the nose. Crap. I cuff the arm bar guy and knock him to the floor. I turn and grab the guy that punched me in the nose and cuff him as well. Now I'm out of cuffs.

Fuck it. I dive in to the next group and end up rolling on the floor with two people. One of the other cops is standing over us with his baton and is jabbing into the pile. The problem is he is hitting me as often as he is hitting anyone else. All three of us fighting stop fighting for a minute. I think for just a second we all thought about kicking the cop with the batons ass.

This scuffling and grappling goes on for about 10 minutes as we drag people, men and women alike, out of the bar into the parking lot. Someone has a handful of tie wraps that we are using for cuffs. The great thing is that not once did a knife or gun come into play. A couple of tables and a random pool cue jumped in the fight but overall it was knuckles.

In the end the band and the bartenders side with the cops and the tide turns. We get all the fighting shrimpers outside and end up with 17 people in cuffs or ties. Everyone in uniform or in cuffs has a bloody nose, split lip or swollen eye. Most of the arrestees are laughing and joking. They had the time of their lives and to be perfectly honest, I had a lot of fun too. It's not very often that you walk away from a full out bar brawl and no one goes to the hospital.

In the end we issued summons to everyone and as we cut them lose they head back into the bar. My favorite moment was when several of the guys came and shook my hand told me good fight and asked if we wanted to come in for a drink. I had to take a raincheck on the drink but told them to schedule the next celebration on a night we were off.

SUNBURN

South Louisiana is home to dozens of oil refineries and they are a major provider to the livelihood of the region but they can be a bit dangerous sometimes.

The Tenneco Refinery had a major explosion and fire in a holding tank around 1979. That one I remember well because I was only three blocks away on a baseball field when it blew. The explosion and shock wave was utterly terrifying. That event took one man's life and made a lasting impression on me.

Ten plus years later, I was working as a medic for the local Sheriff's Office on the rescue squad. My office is again only blocks away from the refinery yard. I would never have believed I would be part of another event there.

The explosion rocks the building. The wave of heat and light was amazing and staggering at the same time. Tiny pieces of metal come floating out of the sky.

The 'cat cracker' had exploded and looked like a giant roman candle as gouts of fire spew from the top of it. As a medic, my first thought was to help the wounded so we rush to the main gate of the refinery to help in the rescue efforts.

They have one patient, a man burned over a large part of his body leaving most of his clothes burned off. The only parts not burned are where his watch and belt are. Most of his burns are 1st and 2nd degree so in that sense he is lucky. We rush him to the hospital and head back to set up a triage area, hoping we don't have to use it. The refinery had a little luck on its side as well. The explosion happens on a Sunday night with just the minimal employees, so we quickly realized there was no one else that needed emergency medical attention. Our skills were needed in a different way. Dozens of fire fighters were battling this blaze and we set up to watch for their health and safety.

I stood at a table and shuttled water to the fireman making sure they were hydrated and keeping an eye on them.

Many hours later as we wrapped up and went back to the station the guys started laughing and asked me if I was alright. I said sure why? "Go look in a mirror." As I step in front of the mirror I am reminded of the scene from Close Encounters of The Third Kind. I am sun burned….on half my face and only one arm. I have stood most of the night with only the right side of my body facing the fire. It made the rest of the week very trying.

~~COUNTRY COME TO TOWN~~

Mardi Gras is such a huge event. It swells the population of the city immensely for that two week period, and especially for the last 4 days heading into Fat Tuesday. Every medic works, every day, during that time. There are no vacations, and it's still barely enough for coverage.

The police are so understaffed that they get assistance. That assistance comes in the form of other departments. The state police send hundreds of extra officers to work the streets. Many other state agencies send manpower to assist as well including the Department of Corrections. They send guards from some of the biggest prisons in the state.

The guards come in from the rural areas that surround the prisons. The world they leave is an extremely controlled environment via the prison systems rules and responsibilities. They are then thrust into the largest street party in the world with all the insanity and debauchery society can muster. Things are bound to go poorly.

My unit is stationed on the corner of Bourbon St. and Toulouse. It is Saturday probably the biggest party day of the Mardi Gras season. The weather is beautiful, the crowd is friendly, and the women are gorgeous and scantily clad. What more could one ask for? Entertainment, that's what.

We share this corner with a trio of guards from Angola State Penitentiary. They have two tasks. General safety and orderliness of this corner and more importantly, to me at least, the ambulance crews protection while we are working on patients. With this in mind, I begin the day by kissing up to them immediately, and sharing our coffee and snacks. My momma may have raised an ugly child, but not a stupid one. These guys could make our life easy or hard and it was up to us to decide which.

There was one thing that was readily apparent with our three country boys. They liked titties.

A lot! Personally, I couldn't blame them. So do I.

The hotel on the corner where we were had several stories worth of balconies and there was always someone on it trying to entice the ladies passing to make a trade with them. For those of you not aware the trade would consist of a view of the woman in questions breast for 3 cents worth of Chinese made plastic beads, but who am I to question commerce. Our three guards would be right up front ogling away.

That being said, they were just a smidgen homophobic, and not at all pleased to see a man expose himself. If ladies on the balcony would convince a man to drop their pants they would go nuts (pun intended). I watched the Sergeant of the group put on his leather gloves, with the lead filled knuckles, and when a penis appeared he grabbed the poor sap by his member and drug him out of the crowd.

The poor sap would be trailing behind his baby maker as if it were a leash. He would be roughly placed against the wall. All of his beads would be confiscated and he would be sent up the street away from the revelers with a warning about what would be done to his privates, if he returned. The show was fabulous. The only thing we were missing was popcorn.

The day wore on with our trio providing loads of entertainment and tons of laughs but as the crowds grew, so did our business. Our normal method for getting to a patient was to travel on foot with all our gear on our stretcher. We would travel away from Bourbon St. by one block, and come back up to

Bourbon at a cross street closest to the call. Over 95% of our calls were on Bourbon (shocking!!). This was because of the volume of people, the sheer sea of humanity that was on Bourbon made it virtually impassable without serious effort or hardship. Our method would take us out of the way but was usually quicker by virtue of being less populated and let's face it, it wasn't as if we couldn't use the exercise.

We receive a radio call of an overdose at a club about a block and a half away from our location. It's now at the height of the crowd size and darkness is upon us. We began stacking our gear on the stretcher so that we could start our hike.

Our new found friends asked what was up, and we filled them in. The leader of this band said that he would lead us and he felt he could make a hole in the crowd. He was sure we could go straight down Bourbon St. to the call. Hell, I was game. What's the worst that could happen?

The three guards arranged themselves in a triangle with the sergeant out front and one on each of our flanks. Ok, I could see how this could work. Sarge stuck his whistle in his mouth and then extended his expandable baton and started moving forward........Oh shit!

He would blow his whistle and whack the shit out of anyone in his way as we moved through the crowd. I think he was making a dozen new patients for us by bludgeoning the crowd. We were kind of towed along in the wake of his whistle and violent acts.

Two thoughts were running through my mind. One was that I thought if my bosses got word of this fiasco, someone was in deep shit, and since that someone was normally me, I was not pleased. The second problem was that they were making more work by beating on the crowd and we were busy enough without the help.

By the end of our Mardi Gras the fun we watched and participated in with our friends from the penal system was worth any extra work they brought us. I am not sure how life back in the sticks was going to live up after a week of beer, breasts and beating the shit out of tourists.

DEEP BREATH

As a Paramedic you have a lot of responsibility on your shoulders when caring for patients. The calm aloof attitude takes a while to settle into, but is needed to render sound patient care. This is even made more difficult when you are friends with the person you're rendering aid to.

Gwen and I had been friends for years. She was a Paramedic also, and we both worked for the city so we had a lot in common. She was a runner and on her day off, she would go out and jog. This day she thinks that when she went out for her run she ran through a cloud of someone spraying their lawn with a pesticide or some similar poison. Whatever it was she was highly allergic to it.

Like most medics she tried to handle it herself first. Most medics despise the thought of calling an ambulance for themselves. It's embarrassing. By the time her daughter had called for help and I had arrived on the scene her condition was getting bad. Her hands were swollen up like cartoon hands, with sausages for fingers. Her face and neck were also swelling causing her to be extremely short of breath.

Her being a Paramedic makes this a pretty unique situation. She understands what's happening, and also knows the treatments that are standard to help her. As soon as I got her in the unit, I was getting her on an airway treatment and starting an IV so that medicine could be administered.

I was sweating bullets. The airway treatment wasn't working. She had already taken Benadryl. Normal course of action says an injection of epinephrine into the muscle. This technique allows the medicine to take its time to move into the system as it is basically synthetic adrenaline and can do as much harm as good if used incorrectly. My fear was that it wouldn't act fast enough. She was truly looking like death on a cracker. I knew if her breathing got any worse, I would need to intubate her (place the tube into her lungs to assist her breathing) and by all that is holy, I did not want to intubate a friend.

    I looked at her and asked her "IV Epi?" She knew just what I was asking. Instead of taking the shot in the muscle I would go with the fastest method possible I would mix a cocktail of Epinephrine to push directly into her IV and into her bloodstream. The upside would be her breathing would improve almost immediately. The downside was that with the already serious strain on her heart, I could kill her with the extra adrenaline.

    She looked me right in the eyes. Her breathing was ragged and she was having to use her shoulders to help her take a deep breath, but there was no doubt in her gaze. She just shook her head yes.

    I quickly drew up the medication and inserted it in her IV. I grabbed her hand and squeezed it just as I pushed the medicine home. She gripped my hand loosely at first, then, as the medicine took hold, she tightened her grip to almost painful levels. I was holding my breath the whole time saying a prayer to the paramedic gods that my gamble wouldn't cost Gwen.

    One of the best sound I've ever heard was at that moment when she suddenly took a deep breath.

~~BOAT ACCIDENT~~ 〰〰〰〰〰〰〰〰〰〰〰〰〰〰〰〰〰

I've said many times that family members are the hardest people to care for. The emotional connection makes doing your job, very, very difficult, but sometimes the choice is not left up to you.

My father had called me and asked if my son and I wanted to go out in the boat. My mom and my two nieces Cheyenne and Gabrielle were all just going for a ride in Lake Pontchartrain. I said sure Blade, my son, would enjoy it.

We all headed to the boat launch at Bonnabel Blvd. Got the boat launched and were getting the kids in to their life jackets. Its early June the weather is hot and beautiful.

We pull away from the dock, and make our way around the break water of the marina. My Father and I are standing at the center console controlling the boat. My Son is sitting in the fishing seat at the bow, with both his cousins sitting behind him on the seat. My Mother is sitting to the port side of the boat with her back to the port so that she can take pictures of the kids as we cruise the lake.

We're headed towards the Causeway Bridge, a 24 mile long twin set of bridges that cross the lake. We want to cross under it and go to an area on the other side to fish with the kids. It's a few miles from the marina to the bridge, and we run in a nice straight line until we get to the bridge. The way the bridge legs are oriented you need to slalom them to get to the other side. We are making our approach and I ease back on the throttle. I turn the wheel to make the move under the second bridge. Nothing happens! The wheel spins freely. In a fraction of a second the options are trying to run through my head. I remember slapping at the throttle hoping to slow us. It's all too late and we impact the bridge pylon just port of center.

In the impact my Son, who is sitting up in the chair, is thrown out of the boat. I see nothing else at that moment but his eight year old body flying out into the water. Before the boat has stopped, I dove out after him. It had nothing to do with training. I can't even say I thought about it. It was not a conscious decision.

He has popped up thanks to his life jacket and was looking a little freaked out. I imagine my face looks the same. I swim to him, and he latches on with vice grip like strength. I'm telling him I got him and start to turn us, to swim back to the boat. He starts fighting me and saying my shoe, my shoe. He will not let me tow him because he sees his Croc floating away. I swim with him and retrieve the shoe and then side stroke to the boat.

I can see my nieces standing near the center console and my father meets us at the stern. I lift my son as best I can, and my dad pulls him up. I'm trying to find footing to get myself in the boat when he tells me my Mother is unconscious.

As I get in the boat I see my Mother crumpled on the deck blood surrounding her head. I have my Father shuffle the kids to the back of the boat they all appear physically fine. My dad is obviously shaken but appears uninjured. As I rush to her side I see that she is bleeding from a large cut on her head but that is not my main concern. My concern is that she is unconscious, and we are in a boat with no steering, floating in the lake. I pull off my shirt and wrap her head to staunch the bleeding and position her so her airway is open and she is breathing regularly.

With all the bad luck that happened that day, we received an amazing piece of good luck at the very moment we desperately needed it. My Father had already dialed 911 and given them the run down, but that wasn't going to help us with our immediate needs. Our luck came in the form of highway maintenance. The thing that on any other day would have had me cursing the delays and problems, was today a blessing. The Highway Department had a vehicle doing work almost directly over where we had drifted. They were a crew set up especially for bridge work and had a hoist on the back of their truck with a lift basket as well as a Jacobs's ladder. My Father was able to get us moving with the trolling motor and finally under the work crew. They had lowered a rope so we could stay in position. They then lowered the basket down to the boat.

 My Mom had regained consciousness by then and was moaning and disoriented. We just talked to her to keep her as calm as possible as we loaded her into the rescue basket. I could see the ambulance arrive above us, and felt very grateful for the men and women of my profession.

 As they hoisted my Mom up in the basket I asked my Dad if he would be okay with the kids, so that I could go with her. He said definitely and went to sit with the kids. He would have to wait for a boat to tow him back to the docks. The ladder was lowered and I climbed up to the roadway above. The road crew were great. They had helped get my mother's basket up and over the rail and had passed her to the medics that were waiting. They wanted to be off further use, so once I was in arms reach they towed me up and over the guard rail.

 At this point I'm shirtless and soaking wet. When I approach the medics and tell them who I am. The normal procedure would be to stick me in the front seat as a passenger and head to the hospital. I didn't know whether either one of them understood when I said I was a medic and that I wanted to assist with her care, but they let me in the back of the unit to help anyway. It had to be the look of desperation on my face.

We took off lights and sirens heading to the trauma center. I had made a quick call to my Wife giving her little detail other than that our son was alright and she needed to meet me at the hospital. As I attempted an IV on my Mom and helped with all the care needed I focused on just the next minute, the next second. Trying desperately to not let my emotions bubble to the surface.

We get to the emergency room. A place I've brought dozens if not hundreds of patients over the years and help rush my mother into the trauma room known as room 4. Surrendering care of a loved one is very hard but my second bit of luck is the Trauma Surgeon and the head nurse on at that very moment were both friends. The nurse had been working at the hospital as long as I'd been a medic and he was a former paramedic that had made quite the name for himself as a trauma surgeon. I gladly let them take over. I found a corner and slid down the wall to gather my thoughts and say a prayer.

My Mother was in a coma for almost a month and over a year later is still dealing with the aftermath of that tragic accident, but I am grateful every day that she is still with us, so that I can tell her I love her and her grandkids have her in their lives.

MORGUE RUN

In my position on the Rescue truck, at the Sheriff's Office, part of our duties included taking corpses to the morgue for autopsy. Definitely not a glamorous part of the job, but a vital one none the less. What was also not uncommon, was when a call such as that was close to shift change, you would try and turf it off onto the next shift coming on. You stalled and sat around until there wasn't enough time to make the run then let them do it after shift change. It wasn't as if it was an emergency.

This tendency to punt it to the other shift set up a particularly interesting scenario. We knew how aggravated the oncoming crew would get about the call right out the gate so they might overlook the underlying prank we would lay.

We decided the plan called for getting one of the day shift partners in on the shenanigans. That left Sam as the focus of our fun. Hmmmm, what would get the most bang for our buck? Un-dead body! Yep that would work.

The Set Up

With about 30 minutes before shift change we laid out a body bag on the stretcher in the unit and Mike got in. I zipped him in but didn't put the straps on him. That was part of our plan.

Now we knew if it was just me, Sam wouldn't buy it. He would get suspicious right away, that's why we recruited his partner. So as Sam pulled up just at shift change the stage was set.

The Build Up

As Sam walked up his partner was reading me the riot act. He was bitching at me for holding over a morgue run that they would have to take at the start of their shift. I dutifully bitched right back and said that my partner and boss Mike had to leave early so it couldn't be helped and to stop whining. This byplay was enough to get Sam in the conversation on his partner's side, which was just what we wanted.

This is where I show contrition and apologize saying, look I know it sucks but we didn't have a choice. I'll come in early tonight if it makes you feel better. This mollified Sam and he went to grab his gear.

The Prank

Sam and his partner jump in the truck with Sam in the passenger seat ready to make the trip into the city to drop off the body. Sam's partner puts the truck in gear and hits the gas with the wheel turned so that the truck lurches sideways. Mike takes this moment to roll off the stretcher onto the floor.

Sam's partner hits the brakes and immediately tears into Sam asking why he didn't check to make sure the body was secured to the stretcher. He tells Sam to get his ass back there and square things away.

Now Sam is a good guy, if not just a little gullible, so at this point, he had the bait in his mouth, and we were about to set the hook.

Sam opens the back doors to the truck. I am standing just 10 feet away asking him what was up, to distract him as much as possible. He reaches down and heaves the body bag up on to the stretcher and prepares to secure it. This is the moment that Mike has been waiting for. He bursts out of the body bag roaring like …well like a soul condemned to a body bag and wanting to get out.

Sam had excellent survival instincts.

He didn't freeze. He didn't hesitate. He ran, and ran, and ran. He came out of the back of the truck looking for all the world like Wyllie Coyote. The only things missing was the cut out in the side of the truck shaped like his silhouette. I swear he had a dust cloud behind him as he ran down the street and around the corner screaming at the top of his lungs.

The After effect

We had to take the unit to go find Sam. He was about three blocks away when we caught up to him. By this time his mind had processed what he had seen and knew he had been punked but since his heart beat hadn't slowed yet and his level of embarrassment was peaked, he just kept walking. We got him back to the station where a laugh was had by all....Okay maybe not all. Sam was still pissed. I'm not sure if Sam ever trusted us after that. I'm pretty sure he refused to go on any morgue runs.

ST. PATRICKS PARADE

Every year for St. Patrick's Day there is a big parade running through the French Quarter. This is what New Orleans does as part of the celebrations. Little shock in that with a well-established Irish American community in town, as well as all those wishing they were Irish for a day we have a parade.

This year tragedy struck in the form of a drunk driver. It seems that riding in the parade was a truck from one of the local alcohol distributors. This truck was decorated for Killian's Red beer and was supposed to be part of the festivities. The driver had been drinking reports later showed.

Someone reached into the cab of his truck and stole the hat off his head. Being mad and drunk further impaired his judgement because his solution was to hit the gas and plow into the crowd. He ended up killing one and injuring thirty eight others. This is truly what we call a mass casualty event and how you deal with such a call, I believe, truly defines your collective skills as an ambulance service.

My unit and the Supervisor on that night, were the first dispatched to the scene. We were told they were getting lots of calls and that they would route more units in to help as we got a better idea of our needs.

We got to the scene or at least as close as we could get at the corner of Bienville and Bourbon St. It was pandemonium. We had injured people on the ground, walking wounded just wandering aimlessly. We needed to get a handle on this and fast. Randy, the Supervisor jumped in immediately and went into the Oyster bar on the corner. He politely told the manager that we needed his restaurant and would they clear all the tables to one side and open up the floor. It was brilliant!

We could funnel the patients into the Oyster bar from the Bourbon St. side and treat them. Then move them out on the Bienville St. side to the side and to the ambulances staged there.

One of the tasks I was given was the coordinating of the routes for the units to enter and line up. Most crews wouldn't even get out of their trucks. They would pull up to the corner. I would strip their truck of any supplies we might need, such as the spine boards, c-collars and bandages. While I was doing that another group would be loading patients that had been deemed serious enough to need transport. On our arrival there had been one seriously injured women that the second unit on scene had taken immediately, due to the severity of her injuries.

I think to an outside observer it must have looked like total bedlam. The oyster bar employees were making ice packs and running around moving tables and chairs. We had people sitting or lying on the floor in various states of treatment. Ambulances were lined up on the side street with the red strobes painting the walls as they moved forward to collect their patients. To us, it was like an orchestra. Every instrument had certain notes to play and when everyone played the right notes it made one seamless piece of music.

In the end we were able to treat or transport nearly 40 people in less than an hour and do so with 4 units 8 medics and 2 supervisors and in the end the City gave the restaurant a commendation for service to the community.

ATTITUDE ADJUSTMENT

Some patients just rub you the wrong way. Some can be rude, mean, stupid, or any combination along this theme but as a professional you do your best not to let it get to you. Sometimes your best isn't good enough.

The call was for a severely intoxicated man who had fallen down. We were three in a truck breaking in a new team member. We arrived, figuring this call should be a piece of cake. Our drunk was as advertised. He was lying on the ground still trying to get whiskey out the bottom of a bottle. It doesn't bode well when, as we walk up to him, he slurs. "Fawk, you are some ugly fawka's." Oh lord, this is going to be interesting. He has a big cut on one arm from broken glass from where he fell. We are trying to bandage him up. He is flailing his arm around flinging blood in every direction. My partners are Andy and Mike. Andy's the rookie and Mike's my regular partner. I can tell that this guy is getting under Mike's skin pretty quick.

We get captain drunk tank off the ground, onto the stretcher and into the unit. He is calling us names and cursing at us although his words are so garbled it sounds like a continuous string of vowels "oui aeuieo aaoiu euaoie......fawkas!!" with the occasional clear cuss word.

I tell Andy to jump in the driver's seat. I'll take the back with Mike. Mike is trying to secure the dressings on the patients arm and just general care when vowel man makes a major faux pas. He spits at Mike.

Mike looks right at me and says "Aren't we still having problems with the power to the back of the truck?" To my knowledge we were not having any problems, but I think I got the real message. I reached up to the panel and tripped the breaker killing the power to the rear of the ambulance. No sooner did darkness fall when a loud WHOMP! WHOMP! WHOMP! Sounded. At which point, I turned the breaker back on, and the Whiskey wrangler was in a stuporous state and it appeared that his nose was oddly shaped now…….

We began our journey to the emergency room and just before we arrived, our not very bright occupant revived. He looked right at Mike and said "Ima beetcha asss you soma bisch!" Oddly enough the power momentarily fluttered again and that loud sound of someone's attitude being adjusted filled the truck. When the lights returned, we were greeted by silence. Well not exactly silent, since our patient made a rather odd snoring sound out of the bulbous appendage in the center of his face.

As we wheeled into the emergency room the ER doc looked at our unconscious patient and said "What the hell happened to him?" Mike's reply was "Fell down. He tripped over a liquor bottle and hit his head against his bad attitude. It knocked him the fuck out.

ROCKING CHAIR CPR

Many times in my world you witness things that are done with all the love and emotion, but some people cannot accept the truth of a situation for what it is. It is at these times compassion and understanding must be at a premium.

I was working as the sprint unit. One man in a car that can race to the scenes and make the decision if more help was needed. I was sent to a residence with the information that CPR was in progress. The caller told dispatch that he had arrived at his mother's house and found her not breathing so had immediately started CPR.

On my arrival, the front door is wide open. Knowing the urgency of this call I head in. As I walk into the living room, I am momentarily taken aback. A man, presumably the caller is on his knees performing CPR, which alone is not what has faltered my step. It's the fact that the person he is doing CPR on is dead. Very dead. Dead as in rigor mortis dead.

From where I stand I can instantly surmise that she died while sitting in her rocking chair. She had obviously still been sitting in it, when her son came in. Her body was frozen in that shape of a person sitting in the chair with their hands on the arm rests. Her back was naturally bowed with age which made the CPR he was doing look grotesquely like he was rocking her as if you would the chair.

I lower all my gear to the floor and walk over to him. I put my hands on the shoulders of this man I've never met and tell him in as soothing a voice as I can muster that it's over. This isn't something he doesn't know. It's something he doesn't want to accept. He is throwing everything he has in to saving his mother something I can truly understand. As I stand there he stops his efforts and begins to weep holding his hands to his face.

It's at times like this that are the hardest for me to handle since emotions are difficult. Actions are easier for me, but it's also the moment when I think I can have the most impact. Callousness or cold professionalism at this point will not help this man mourn. One man allowing another to show his feelings and be supportive can change the rest of his life. Once he is able to stand, I take him to the kitchen and he tells me about his Mother.

I have no point of reference for his stories but understanding is not what's needed right now. I'm just a sounding board. I help make the arrangements so the funeral home can come get his Mother and I stay as long as I am able. I hope that the kindness I showed made a difference.

MANNEQUIN MANIA

It is amazing how one item can cause so much trouble. The item I'm referring to was a Halloween decoration that had been confiscated from some kids. They had stolen it, and a bunch of other items and when they were caught by the police, it was all brought back to the station where we were.

Now the first prank was really just a warm up, it would give us ideas which is such a bad thing to have when at work. One of the deputies put the dummy in the back of the patrol car and then called the jail on the radio. He was kind of a psycho so we knew this would get interesting. He told the jail he was coming in with a violent subject in his car and to have people with restraints waiting to help.

He told us to get a good vantage point to watch and took off around the block in his unit. As he approached the gate into the jail, he turned on his lights and kept hitting his siren, giving a serious impression of agitation and urgency. He wheeled into the lot where the jail deputies were all waiting and slammed on the brakes coming to an abrupt stop. He jumped from the car, to open the back door, and yelled into the back seat to calm down. He was amazing. I was starting to believe him, and I knew he was full of shit.

He dove in and started wrestling with the chunk of Halloween decoration. I nearly pissed my pants. While he is flipping, flopping and throwing punches in the back of the car, the jailers are all edging closer and closer. In one last grand dive he flings himself and his pseudo prisoner out of the car, on to the ground and begins bashing its plastic skull into the ground.

The crowd is immediately taken aback. They are at once seized with thoughts of collusion and conspiracy. They will have to choose sides and the fear is immediately seen in their eyes. The Deputy ends his charade by wrapping his arms around the mannequin and planting a kiss on it, followed by his braying laughter. This, at first, confused, then pissed off, the guards, who realized they had been duped. It was a vision of things to come.

With the first act at a conclusion and everyone (OK mostly everyone) finding it extremely humorous, the prevailing thought was, of course, what could we do to top it?

Someone, and I believe I have blocked out which someone as a protective measure, thought it would be a wonderful idea to place the 'body' under someone's car and tell the owner that they ran over a person. That seemed reasonable. But whose car should we put it under? This would be the point when we veered off the rails a bit.

We shared the building, which was an old hospital, with the parishes battered women's shelter, and the person that ran the shelter was someone we knew well enough and she showed up every morning in her Cadillac.

The plan was that, as soon as she got there, the dummy would be placed under her car, cover what was exposed with a sheet, and then call her out to prank her. It got a little out of hand. It was decided, it would look more official if we pulled the ambulance around and left it there with the lights on, then a patrol guy volunteered to put his car there as well. Lastly a friend of our from New Orleans Police was having coffee with us and he said he would put his unit there and do the talking as if it happened in his jurisdiction. Yes, this was getting way out of hand.

Six A.M. comes. The Caddy has arrived and now our stage is set. Everyone takes their places. Our NOPD friend goes in and asked her to step out by the car. As soon as she comes out she sees the set of shoes poking out from under a sheet which is tucked up under her rear tire. She is told, that witnesses saw her hit a pedestrian and drag him away under her car. She towed him for miles never realizing what she did.

This was supposed to be the point where we went...got ya!!... and everyone have a jolly laugh. That is not what occurred. When she saw the body she froze and when she was told what we claimed happened, she broke down. She let out a shrill cry, almost a scream and ran back to her office and locked the door. We immediately cleaned up the evidence and hauled ass leaving one poor bastard to knock on her door and apologize.

While hiding away, trying to act innocent, we were summoned to the Administration building. Oh crap. All of the culprits from the event were assembled including the NOPD Officer. We were ushered into an office, oh shit, this was the Sheriff's Office. We stood in front of the desk. The look on his face was one of acute displeasure. He looked at all of us then he said "I'm guessing you retards were unaware that the person you pulled the prank on this morning is my cousin?" Oh craptastic.

Sergeant Morris Cavaliere, Jr. A friend. I first met Mo when we were both working as medics, and had the pleasure to move in and out of the same circles he did. We had similar backgrounds having both been cops and medics. We shared a passion for teaching others our skills and had occasion to do so several times a year. Our paths crossed at work on occasion, as I was working as a medic for the city and he was a motorcycle officer.

It was a beautiful Sunday and I was working with Cesar, one of the best medics I knew. We were hanging out on St. Charles Avenue just cruising around looking at pretty girls. We got one of those calls that cause a chill to run up your spine.

Officer down.

The call was a for a motorcycle officer hit by a car on Napoleon Ave. We were just blocks away. As we raced to the scene we got our game plan together on how we would attack the call. We had worked together long enough that not a lot of words were needed. It was like dancing with a frequent partner. You knew all their moves and complimented each other.

The view through the window was telling. The Police Harley was mangled and the Officer was face down in the street well past where the bike had stopped. We bailed out of the truck at a run going into our battle plan, grabbing our gear and meeting at our patient. He was facedown wearing his helmet so we prepped his back and rolled him onto a spineboard.

It was Mo! Someone we both knew very well. Cesar and I have the very briefest of eye contacts but a galaxy of information passes between us. We are shocked by who it is and saddened, but we have to go above and beyond with our care. We get Mo packaged up and loaded into the unit. Cesar looks at me again, and says "I got him." His meaning is clear one of us has to drive the other has to tech the call and he has stepped up and said he wants to be in the back with Mo. All these years later I am both grateful and pissed at Cesar for that.

Before we pull away from the scene I had called dispatch and told them we would be heading to the trauma center and to let NOPD know we are hauling ass with one of their own.

NOPD are always there for their own. Before we hit the first turn we had two police cars running lights and sirens in front of us with one behind as we approached red lights, other units had taken up position shutting down traffic to give us a non-stop run to the hospital. The allegiance they showed to their brother in blue was awe inspiring.

We had called ahead and given the hospital a report. We told them it was an Officer and a friend. As we pull onto the hospital ramp the doctors and nurses from the ER are waiting outside for us. They take Mo from us and rush, with speed and purpose, into the hospital. The helpless feeling afterward is harder than when we had a task to do.

It doesn't take them long to tell us that it's bad. His head injury is extremely serious and they are taking him to surgery. It was the last time I ever saw Mo, and a moment I frequently think about when contemplating my own frailty.

KNEE DEEP GAMBLE

    I have been known to take some chances. Gamble when making a decision, especially when working. I tend to land on the high risk, high reward side of the equation. Trouble with that mind set is you can't win all the time, sometimes your plan will sink you, literally.

    I was working one of my part-time jobs for a New Orleans area private Ambulance service. It was a nasty wet and dreary day. We were sent to a local facility that provided long term care for people with the need for specialized treatment, such as respirators.

    Our patient was in need of just such a tool. We were transferring her to the hospital for some treatment or other, so she would need to be on our portable battery powered ventilator with our bottled oxygen attached. Our transport would take us across town to the hospital, but as we set off the weather had intensified and was making the travel very difficult. It was taking us a long time to navigate safely around areas that were flooding.

    We arrived just outside the hospital to find a serious problem. The ambulance entrance to the hospital was on an elevated ramp basically a second floor area. The problem was the street in front of the hospital was a lake. We would have to push through 3 to 4 feet of water to enter the ramp. Crap.

    We sat within sight of the ER doors watching the rain and monitoring our patient trying to come up with an alternative. Dispatch said the rain wasn't stopping. The water wasn't going down, if anything, it was rising. We had another problem we only had so long on the portable ventilator. Its battery could be charged but the amount of oxygen we had on hand was quickly running low.

    I came to a decision. I won't say it was a good one but right or wrong I've lived by the motto that it's better to make a decision and do something than do nothing and let fate decide for you. I was going to see how much water this truck could handle.

    I called the ER and told them we were going to try and get up their ramp if they could be ready to help us with oxygen to swap over to. They stated they would be waiting for us. I had my partner sit with our patient and I would drive. Hell, it was my idea no sense both of us getting into shit for this.

    I started off slow, but saw quickly that it was very deep. I changed my tactic. I thought speed would be better, and yes, I am an idiot. If I was smart I wouldn't have so many interesting stories to tell.

    I hit the gas sending a cresting wave out in front of the truck. We hit the ramp and I started up! I thought I had it made when the engine sputtered and died. I coasted a few more feet and watched our wave out pace us. That's when my partnered hollered that we were taking on water.

    Well, no choice now. I jumped out of the truck and landed in water only about knee deep but as I made my way towards the back doors the water kept creeping up. I got to the back door at navel depth and figured this was going to be interesting. I opened the doors to see 3 or so inches in the back of the truck. I'm pretty sure it was never intended to function this way. I unlatched the stretcher and began to roll it out figuring once the wheels locked the bed would be just over the water line. I just made it.

    My partner and I had another problem when we began to move the stretcher we couldn't see where the wheels were and the last thing we wanted was to hit a hole and dump our patient into the water. Our solution was to lift the stretcher and carry it until we could roll it. All this did was shove us deeper into the water as we moved along.

We finally got our patient to dry land and could look back down at our sunken unit. That's when we notice the news cameras that filmed my recreation of the sinking of the titanic. Dripping wet and thoroughly dejected we entered the Emergency Room to the applause of the staff as they had watched us through the window. They kindly took over care of our patient and got us some scrubs so that we could have dry clothes.

I called dispatch to tell them what was up, but they had obviously been watching the news and already knew. What a shock. I was in trouble again.

THE BIBLE AND BODY GREASE

There are a lots of weird shit that goes on in New Orleans, so it takes a lot to shock or befuddle me. So, it was a bit perplexing to see a naked man holding a Bible above his head, and preaching in front of Richard's, the diner my partner and I were going to for breakfast. To make things even more surreal as we got out the truck and headed towards him he looked as though he glistened.

We were getting off shift in less than 30 minutes this was not what we wanted to deal with. We called dispatch told them what we had, and asked for the police to assist, just to make sure we covered our bases, and proceeded to approach our new patient, to see exactly what form of mental defect he was experiencing.

He was standing outside the diner preaching the New Testament at the top of his lungs. He was naked, barefoot, and crazy as a shithouse rat. We stepped up and attempted to talk to him but he was not giving us the time of day. I guess we were interfering with his sermon. I reached out and grabbed him by the forearm to turn him toward me and he jerked back. He was slick with oil or lotion from head to toe. He was as slippery as a Louisiana politician on Election Day.

This was going to be interesting. I'd heard of chasing a greased pig but never thought I'd do it, much less chase a greased naked crazy man. Well here goes nothing. I wrap both hands around his arm to guide him to our truck that's when he lunged away and POP! His arm popped right out of my hands.

This would be the point where the naked crazy man with the Bible started running……….

Well I am not a little guy or a skinny guy and running is kinda against my religion, so we needed another way. I know, we will chase him with the ambulance! I get in the driver's seat and take off after him. He is making this too easy I think, as I watch him run down the middle of the street. My partner has his door open and has one foot out on the running boards. So I head right out after our quarry and line him up with the passenger door. As I bring him alongside, my partner, stands up and prepares to grab him. He kind of dives at our runner and slides right off of him. He then proceeds to bounce twice on the asphalt. Oops!

Crazy man decided to zig off through a parking lot away from us at this point. Running right toward the NOPD Officers that hadn't got the memo "Slippery when Wet" so they tried to tackle him. He went down but not before they went skidding of crashing into each other. This impersonation of keystone cops (and medics) went on for a good 10 minutes by this time my partner was thoroughly annoyed, He was dirty, greasy, and had scrapes on both hands and elbows from planting them on the asphalt. He was insistent that we get him. Our human slip and slide ran around a building and we headed with the truck to cut him off at the pass. We got there just as he emerged.

Up to now it had been like chasing an NFL wide receiver and then trying to tackle a stick of butter. My partner had finally had enough. As we got alongside him again the unit door flung open knocking our man and his bible to the pavement. That was all it took because everyone descended on him. It was dog pile time. It is the only time in my career I have ever brought a patient into the ER naked, greased, and now hog tied. It made for an interesting report to write.

SEIZURE SOLUTION

Let's talk about people that fake seizures. There are a lot of them out there that do this. Whether it's for attention or....well hell, what other reason would you have to fake a seizure, other than the attention? Some people do it with more success than others. It's all about your level of commitment to your thespian art. I have seen the weak attempt of fluttering eyes and flopping arms and am never impressed. People that do that normal just get barked at to cut that shit out and get the hell up.

Then there are the pros. The ones that have honed their skills to fool the most hardened medic. I know of a particular TROLL that will not even hesitate to piss his own pants, in an attempt to convince you. That's dedication!

Then there are the academy award winners. These are very rare, and to be truthful I have only known one. He will utterly refuse to break character, to the point where you are doubting yourself, on a diagnosis of faking it. This guy was a legend but as all legends do, he met his match. One day he got a particular paramedic on the scene that had been waiting for this very moment.

He had his seizure like fit in front of a Burger King with a full crowd of on lookers. The first step with any of these types of calls is to get them away from their fans, the endearing crowd. Once in the back of the truck all his clothes were cut off. Being the pro that he was he didn't flinch. Once naked our medic ascended to levels of myth, by taking a large needle and sticking our pro right in the scrotum!

Our TROLL screamed. He flew straight up off the stretcher yelling *goddamnsonofabitchinbastardmotherfuckers!!!!!!*

"It's a miracle, he's cured." Responds our paramedic.

The best part is, all you had to do in the future, was whisper in his ear that you would call the nut stabbing medic, and he would stop, get up and walk away.

~~CRACKERS~~ ⁓⁓⁓⁓⁓⁓⁓⁓⁓⁓⁓⁓⁓⁓⁓⁓⁓⁓⁓⁓⁓⁓⁓⁓⁓⁓

    Its late evening on a weekday when dispatch gives us a call behind the donut shop. It's odd because it's a welfare check on a vehicle. The lady that works the counter at the donut shop says, that every morning, she has a customer that parks his delivery truck in the back of the shop. He came in that morning and had his coffee and when she looked out back late this evening his vehicle was still there. She called because she thinks it has been there all day.

    We arrive and circle around back. There parked against the back fence is a panel van. It is marked with a local cracker and cookie company logo. The hood is cold so it's been here awhile. The back doors are locked but I'm able to jimmy a small vent window on the front of the van and am able to get the door open to go in. The pass through from the cab to the back of the van is blocked by a wall of boxes filled with crackers. It's very dark inside, so I have a small flashlight that I hold in my mouth as I search around. My light rests on a body from behind. It is sitting up on boxes and leaning against a shelf. I place my hand on the shelf to stabilize myself and feel something wet under hand. I turn the light in that direction and find I have placed my hand on a tongue.

    I am staggered by this for a moment, but with one hand held away from my body I work my way to the back doors and open them. As I shed light in the truck, I can now see the trucks owner with a shotgun wound to the face. At least now the tongue makes sense.

    With lights shined in, it is a horror story. There is blood, bone, and brain everywhere. All the boxes are peppered with it. It is a gruesome scene that we must tend to. My partner and I take the man to the morgue, while crime scene handles the truck.

    The rest of our night was busy so we put the call from our minds. In the morning, I had to drop off something in the Detective bureau. I find the detectives sitting around eating cookies and crackers. They offer me some. I politely decline.

PARA GRAVIDA

I think the general public would be amazed at how many children are delivered in the field. I am a light weight having delivered only 9 (not counting my own kids). Para gravida is the medical term we use to determine number of live births (para) and number of pregnancies (gravida). We are trained for normal births and a few types of emergency but sometimes the calls are enough to push our training and our nerve to the limits.

The call is for a woman in labor. The name of my partner and the young Tulane student that rode as our volunteer that night has long faded from memory but I remember the details of the call very well.

We head to the residence with lights and sirens since we are told the patients contractions are very close together. When we arrive at the front door it's open and we head on in. Our patient is sitting on the sofa and tells us her water has broken and that she is having contractions two minutes apart. Crap that's close together and she seems very knowledgeable.

I ask her how many times she has been pregnant (gravida) she tells me 11 times. In my brain I am saying holy crap! When I ask how many children she has had she tells me 10, with two miscarriages that makes one of the pregnancies twins. Oh peachy.......

There is a known fact, when it comes to pregnancies, which is almost always true. The more times someone is pregnant the faster the baby comes when the birthing begins. This did not lend to good news for us. It meant we had a choice, stay and deliver the baby at the house, or pray to the blessed mother of acceleration and race for the hospital. We decide on speed. It's the best option because the house is full of people, mostly kids, and I don't want to perform for an audience.

We get her on the stretcher and into the truck. Now it's time to take a look at things. I get down and ask her to open her legs, so I can examine her. We are just pulling from the curb, and what I see causes me to yell to the driver to step it up. She has a prolapsed cord. What that means is there is pressure on the cord cutting off circulation to the baby. Crap! The volunteer is in the back with me so I turn to her and take off my watch and hand it to her. She looks at me odd, not sure why I was doing.

I tell her what I am about to do and she looks at me in horror. I have her move toward the patients head to talk to her and keep her calm. I have to insert my hand into the women to lift pressure off the cord. That would be why I took off my watch. It had been a gift.

Now I have delivered a lot of babies in the field in my years and transported countless pregnant women but I have never had to put my hand in a patient's vagina. This is a first on the job. I'm trying to start my IV with one hand and with my volunteers help. I have her call the hospital and then relay what's happening. I am told to head straight upstairs to the delivery rooms.

We get to the hospital and I have a sheet over the patient and my arm as we get the stretcher out I am walking along side continually holding the pressure off the cord and trying to reassure my patient. I try to hand over my task but the staff just usher me onward.

We get in the elevator and have one of those really strange moment, when we are all standing there listening to the music and waiting to get to the floor, it felt surreal. As we get off on the delivery floor the team of doctors and nurses are waiting for me and take the patient the stretcher and me into the delivery room. I am finally relieved of my duties and allowed to leave so that they can do an emergency C-section.

I am no sooner cleaned up and sitting down to complete the report when the doctor comes out of the delivery room. She makes eye contact with me and shakes her head. Damn, I didn't want to hear that. He tells me that the cord was prolapsed for a while and that there was nothing I could do. None of that makes me or my team feel any better. Life in EMS doesn't allow for you to think too long on the tragedies. We must head on to our next call.

CODE AND CACCIATORE

My partner and I were called to a scene that the police were already on. It seems a dispute between neighbors was going on and one of the parties wasn't feeling very well. It's a beautiful summer evening close to sunset and everyone is on the front lawn as we pull up. One of the onlookers is a tow truck driver that we know because he is in EMT school.

Our patient is sitting in a lawn chair he is a heavy set guy in his fifties and even from a distance I can tell his blood pressure must be through the roof. He is flush and I can see his temple and jugulars bulging out.

It seems that his son and a neighbor had gotten in a fight, and he had chased the guy away. He had just finished a huge dinner of chicken cacciatore and ran a few blocks definitely not a healthy choice.

As we stood there and checked our patients' blood pressure the situations got much worse, much faster than we were ready for. Our patient began to have a seizure falling from his chair right into my arms. We have him on the monitor and can clearly watch as he goes into v-fib. He is in cardiac arrest on the front lawn in front of the neighborhood. Crap.

A witnessed arrest, meaning you watched someone die, is not all that common. It's one of those times when you have seen the Reaper pull someone away from you, and you want to give every ounce you have to drag them back and give the Reaper the finger.

We start to scramble. Getting CPR going and attempting to intubate our patient. We defibrillate our patient and get him back! We race him on to the stretcher and into the truck. This is going to be a juggle, and we need help.

As you're probably aware, normally one partner drives and the other techs the call in the back, and on occasion you might get a fire fighter or a volunteer in the back helping out. This day that option isn't available to us so Louie, my partner, and I take a little more unique approach.

We grab our friend the tow truck driver and stick him behind the wheel. Is this allowed? No. Is it a good idea? Probably not. Are we in a tight spot and doing it anyway? You bet your ass.

We get him up front because he doesn't have any patient care experience and we need a lot done but he knows how to drive. We think. He drives a tow truck. What could go wrong? Well pretty much everything.

Our driver, we find out, has no concept of subtle. He hits the gas and it's all the way to the floor. It's like medical care in a Tilt-A-Whirl. We are bashing around continuing our care when it gets worse. Our patient codes again! We start CPR again. Drugs, shocks and Oxygen not necessarily in that order. We are making corners and its rocking and rolling in the back, bad.

At some point in our adventure the next bit of bad shows up. After prolonged CPR a lot of air gets pushed into the stomach, this can result in the patient vomiting, and yes that's exactly what happens! Chicken Cacciatore is bubbling out of our patient. It is bright red and the smell is acidic and putrid at the same time with the undercurrent of tomato.

Louie is leaning over the patient trying to suction his mouth clear while I am doing CPR. As I watch his face he is retching. It is a strong dry heave that looks like it is starting in his back and working its way up and over his head. Now I was doing well up to this point, pretending I couldn't smell it. Now that I see Louie I think it's like a yawn and is contagious.

I start feeling that spasmodic feeling in my belly, and my throat is constricting, and I just know I'm gonna ralph if I don't get some clear (clean fresh) air. I open the side door of the unit and let it swing to the side. A little air gets in but with just the side its pushing it into the cab and now our tow truck driver is making barfing sounds.

The only thing I can think of between CPR and retching is to open the back doors. So I swing them wide and feel a welcome draft cut through the cab for the last few blocks into the hospital.

We get to the ER ramp with all our doors swinging open and both medics and our driver green. We race in with our patient, and hand them off to the staff. We are absolutely no help as we run out to the scrub sink and vomit our guts up. The smell Chicken Cacciatore still makes me queasy all these years later.

~~AFTERWARD~~

Thank you for reading my rambling adventures. I hope you enjoyed reading them as much as I did telling them. I warned you that I would take you for a ride emotionally so I hope it was good for you.

Now if you bought this book electronically I would be truly grateful if you'd go and leave a **review**. Be honest, I'm a big boy I can take it. The more reviews I get the better the book's exposure is and I need all the exposure I can get…. hmmm maybe that's not exactly what I meant.

Also please go to Facebook and the books website and leave a comment and/or share the page with your friends. That way you'll be the first to hear about any future projects!

Finally, I hope you got a smidgen of insight into the life of your average public servant so give them a big thank you next time you see them.

B.J. Schneider

October 2015

www.xiphosbooks.net

Don't miss the next exciting collection from B.J. Schneider

February 2016

A Salty Life & A Traitors Death

..It's tough being a modern day pirate

Hannibal "Salty" Greco is a smuggler, a brigand, and a 21st century rogue but his loyalty to those close to him is his best asset.

August 2016

Welcome to New Orleans... The life the save may take your own.

This is the follow up to Welcome to New Orleans How Many shots did you hear. This collection broadens our look including public service with stories from EMS, Police and other great moments in and around the city of New Orleans

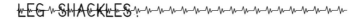

SNEEK PEEK

The following is a story from Volume 2 of the short story collection.

Welcome to New Orleans... The life the save may take your own.

LEG SHACKLES!

When I look back on things I've done as my younger self, I realize how dumb I was, or at the very least how it looks to me in the rear view mirror. This story is about one of those little things that quickly became less little.

As a father that was divorced, I had my daughter with me on every other weekend. We had a lot of fun together and I think with a little help from me she has grown up to be an amazing person (I'm of course probably bias......).

The problem was as a part-time parent I will admit to having difficulty with certain aspects. Things such as child proofing my apartment. Hell it wasn't even adult proofed.

I was working as a policeman at the time and had all the typical cop paraphernalia around. I was extremely cautious when it came to my firearms, but much less so when it came to other tools of the trade. My daughter would routinely play with my hand-cuffs, listening to the clickity, click as she closed them and watching how they folded up on the chain.

I didn't think much about this. It was the early 90s and I was a child of the era that the only bad toy was one you choked on, other than that it was fair game.

The day that changed that thought process was the day she got a hold of a set of leg shackles. Now for those of you not in the know. Leg shackles are slightly larger than hand-cuffs, with a significant longer chain so that someone wearing them can shuffle along while wearing them.

I was in the kitchen doing who knows what since I didn't cook. Hell, my cabinets didn't have food. They had the pieces of a late 70s Harley Davidson I was rebuilding. I hear my daughter playing in the next room and then the sound of her walking. She is three or four at the time, so I look to see what she is up to and she comes into the room with one leg shackle secured around her neck. The other is dragging on the ground behind her like the end of a leash!

I have been shot at, stabbed, rushed into burning buildings but never to my recollection panicked.... until right then. I ran over to her and sure enough the latch had secured and the only way to get them off was a key.

A key. That shouldn't be a problem. I'm a cop. I have two pair of hand-cuffs on my duty belt. A handful more in my trunk. I had a key on my key ring, one on my duty belt and an emergency one in my wallet. There was just one small, minor problem.

THE KEYS DIDN'T WORK!!

It seems that when I made the trade for the leg shackles, I failed to check and see if they were the same key. I just ASSUMED. We all know what that will get you. My panic level increased. What the hell should I do? I tried prying on them to pop them open. All that did was cause them to get even tighter.

I call a cop, friend, that lives close by. He doesn't have a key that works. I call dispatch and they get a road unit on the air and they don't have a key. I have visions of listening to my daughter scream and cry, while I take a hack saw to the cuff around her neck.

I am finally able to find someone with a key. It's the jail (of course), which is eight miles away. A unit from the jail runs lights and sirens down to my house to help me get the shackle free from her neck.

All this time my daughter wants the damn thing off of her. The funny thing is <u>she</u> didn't panic. I was doing enough of that for both of us.

In the end she was safe. I was happy for her, and embarrassed for me. It was a lesson that I've always remembered. Always think through the possibilities. Oh, and don't play with leg shackles.

...................For more great stories make sure to check out this book and others by B.J. Schneider

About the Author

B.J. Schneider is the author of 'Welcome to New Orleans…How many shots did you hear?' and A Salty Life & a Traitor's Death, as well as being a Paramedic, Police Officer, Safety Manager and occasional adventurer (He never knew what he wanted to be when he grew up).

He is also the owner and president of XIPHOS BOOKS & TRAINING where he helps market his books as well as offering quality training in safety, Tactical medicine and various other areas.

He lives in the New Orleans area with his wife Rose his grown daughter Brittanie and his son Blade (Luna the boxer says hi to!). To contact him please go to

www.xiphosbooks.net

Or email him at:

contact@xiphosbooks.net

or

xiphosbooks@gmail.com

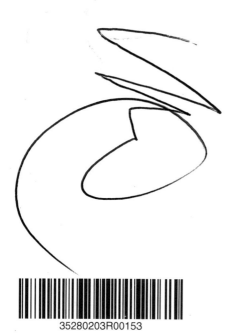

Made in the USA
San Bernardino, CA
20 June 2016